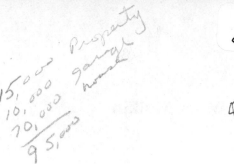

Aerobic Walking

The Weight-Loss Exercise

Other books by Mort Malkin

Psyching Up for Tennis

Data—Matter—O, Poetry and Science

Walking: The Pleasure Exercise

Aerobic Walking

The Weight-Loss Exercise

A Complete Program
to Reduce Weight, Stress, and Hypertension

Mort Malkin

John Wiley & Sons, Inc.
New York • Chichester • Brisbane • Toronto • Singapore

Copyright © 1995 by Mort Malkin
Published by John Wiley & Sons, Inc.

Library of Congress Cataloging-in-Publication Data

Malkin, Mort.
    Aerobic walking : the weight-loss exercise : a complete program to reduce weight, stress, and hypertension / Mort Malkin.
       p.   cm.
    Includes index.
    ISBN 0-471-55672-6 (paper)
    1. Walking—Health aspects.   2. Reducing exercises.   3. Stress management.   4. Hypertension—Exercise therapy.   I. Title
RA781.65.M35   1995
613.7'176—dc20.   94-40817

Printed in the United States of America.
10 9 8 7 6 5 4 3 2 1

Acknowledgments

In the worlds of health and exercise we learn from those we treat and teach, just as they learn from us. I have learned not only from *Gray's Anatomy* and the papers published in such journals as *The New England Journal of Medicine* and *The Physician and Sportsmedicine,* I have learned from the many participants in the aerobic walk training programs that I have taught. I have observed how they learned, what motivated them, how rapidly they could progress, and what wondrous results they achieved as they reached aerobic levels. I am indebted to them all.

I am grateful to Charles Gerras, the senior editor of my first book in this new/old discipline of walking as preventive medicine. He is a rare individual who saw so early that walking was *the* public health model of exercise.

I thank Abby Drucker, my research assistant and colleague in wellness, for her generous efforts in organizing the hundreds of references that were so important in shaping this book.

I wish also to thank you, my readers, who are going to create a nation of attractive, healthy people.

Contents

Introduction

Health and beauty walk hand in hand. Both are heightened by aerobic walking. With this exercise you will become slimmer and healthier. The positive esthetic and health changes that occur with aerobic walking are brought about by improvements in the body's metabolism. With such metabolic gains, your body can better control blood pressure, blood sugar, calcium exchange, brain chemistry, and how fat or lean you are.

Any exercise that is meant to reduce size and increase health must conform to the definition of a true aerobic exercise, that is, an exercise that uses large muscle groups in an uninterrupted, rhythmic, repetitive, submaximal fashion. The exercises that use the large muscles of the lower body are generally good aerobic exercises. They include running, walking, skating, cross-country skiing, rope jumping, stair climbing, rowing, cycling, and swimming. Aerobic dance and belly dancing, if performed vigorously, also qualify. Those exercises that are fully weight bearing have been observed to be more effective in bringing about metabolic change.

Of all the aerobic exercises, walking has the most advantages. It is safe, inexpensive, convenient, suitable for both athletes and nonathletes, requires no special skills to begin, and needs no special equipment or facilities. The disadvantage of walking is that it is only modestly aerobic. Ordinary brisk walking employs mostly the calf muscles for the power of forward motion. Aerobic walking with the Malkin Technique uses the whole leg for power. Virtually all the muscles of the lower body participate. The total muscle mass is exceptionally large, resulting in greater metabolic change and significant improvement in health and appearance. Using the large muscle groups for power also increases your walking speed, and that

1

ability gives you a sense of self-confidence that extends beyond walking. In addition to power, the smoothness of the technique makes aerobic walking the safest of exercises by minimizing the vertical forces on the joints of the body at every stride. Optimal technique can improve your health and enhance your appearance in as little as eight weeks.

In the pages that follow, I will explain the Malkin Technique—why it works, how to do it, and how to use the Eight-Week Program to lose weight and keep it off forever.

The Weight-Loss Connection. Aerobic walk training will:

o Work in partnership with a weight-loss diet, preventing the loss of lean tissues while accelerating fat loss
o Ensure maintenance of weight loss
o Burn calories and keep your metabolic rate higher for several hours afterward
o Lower your set point (the point at which your weight seems to settle naturally, given your usual diet and activity level)
o Avoid the depression associated with very low-calorie diets

The Health Connection. Aerobic walking will:

o Reduce high blood pressure
o Improve blood lipid profile (high and low density lipoproteins, total cholesterol, and triglycerides) and reduce the risk of coronary heart disease
o Reduce and stabilize blood sugar levels in diabetics
o Improve respiratory function
o Increase immunity
o Reverse the degenerative changes of the aging process.
o Slow postmenopausal loss of calcium from bones
o Quicken thought processes
o Improve self-image and strengthen self-esteem
o Help to prevent depression and anxiety
o Raise energy level
o Strengthen lower back muscles and abdominal muscles

The Keys to Reducing. Three keys to successful reducing are:

1. **Diet.** The deprivation diets practiced today would make even a citizen of ancient Sparta unhappy, and so I offer two chapters, "The Aerobic Diet Guide for Reducing" and "The Aerobic Diet Guide for Maintenance." The two diets are not far apart, which tells you that the *Diet for Reducing* has few limitations. Both diets offer a wide variety of foods and include many hints to help you prepare tasty dishes.

2. **Exercise.** Exercise works synergistically with diet to produce weight loss. For maintaining that loss, exercise is even more critical. The metabolic change that exercise brings about will result in less fat storage. In addition, exercise will keep your appetite in balance with your new weight.

3. **Motivation.** A positive attitude will motivate you to keep both diet and exercise in focus. The chapter on motivation, "Heads, You Win," contains 19 strategies that work.

———

You can become slim and stay slim, notwithstanding the gremlins of heredity. All you need is a simple integrated approach, with aerobic walking providing that all-important ignition spark.

CHAPTER 1

Looking Good
That Special Essence

Is an attractive figure measured in pounds, in inches, or by shape?

My long-time friend, Lorraine, knows that the definitions of fat and slim often depend on who does the defining. She is 5' 1" and weighs, in her words, somewhat over 100 pounds. No one asks her to define *somewhat*.

Lorraine says, "I'm not really fat; I'm just too short for my size." She believes that the measures of weight, size, and shape are interrelated.

Most reducing programs are called weight reduction programs, and people generally set goals of losing a certain number of pounds. Although they say they are interested in weight, they are probably more concerned about size—size of waist, size of thighs, and so on. As they lose a number of pounds and inches, they gain a new focus—how they will look in the new styles of swimwear next summer. They have found a third important reason for reducing: shape.

Shape is not just a matter of slimness. There are slim people who have flabby tissues, a bit of a pot belly, and a less than vigorous overall appearance. There are other slim people who have well-shaped arms and legs, flat abdomens, and radiant vitality. Much of the difference is in the tone of the muscles. Strong muscles have a pleasing spindle shape; flaccid muscles are flat, band-like, and unattractive. Dieting can help you lose weight and inches, but only when you add exercise will you have an admirable shape. Go for muscle tone. Today, lean and strong is considered healthy and beautiful. This ideal body is reflected in the way models and athletes look.

4

How Aerobic Walking Improves Your Looks

There are other dimensions to beauty that go beyond weight, size, and shape. How you stand, how you move, and that elusive quality called *presence* all contribute to the impression you make. Let's look at six fundamentals of the whole esthetic picture—weight, size, shape, posture, grace, and presence—in more detail.

Weight

Imagine two weight extremes—a 300-pound individual of average height and a 90-pound person of the same height. There would be no question about who is fat and who is skinny. Between these extremes, however, height-weight ratios are not always reliable indicators of the image an individual projects.

Weight is not only a function of size—both height and girth—it is also a function of how much of the body is fat and how much is lean tissue. The lean tissue of the body is for the most part made up of the organs (liver, kidneys, brain, and so forth) and the musculoskeletal system (muscles, bones, ligaments, and so forth). Lean tissue is heavier than fat.

If you compare two people of the same *weight*, the one who has strong muscles and little fat will look smaller than the one who has less muscle and more fat. If you compare two individuals of the same *size,* the one who has more muscle mass and less fat will be heavier. Thus, a 5'9" football running back may weigh 200 pounds but should be considered lean.

An investigation reported by Claude Bouchard and his team at Laval University in Quebec provides further insight into how complex the relationship between weight and size can be. In overfeeding experiments, those subjects who gained more weight on a given high caloric diet gained more fat than lean tissue. Those who gained less weight for the same caloric intake, gained it more in lean tissues. The high gainers gained not only more weight, but more size *per pound.* A pound of fat takes up more space than a pound of lean tissue.

Why do we still believe the scale is a mirror of how we look? For most of us, small differences in weight—one or two pounds—

may not indicate fat gain or loss. We must not allow such insignificant differences to cause us unwarranted elation or dejection. Elation should be saved for longer-lasting positive results. Conversely, depression following a small amount of weight gain could be wasted emotion if we lose one or two pounds the next week.

Size

Although better than weight as a measure of body esthetics, size has its shortcomings, too. Waist size is a good example. A 22-inch waist on a 5'3" woman looks great. A 22-inch waist on a 5'7" frame is not healthy. Measurements must be relative to height and body frame.

You should also measure dimensions other than waist size. Chest, hips, thighs, midriff, abdomen (below the waist), upper arms, and neck all contribute to appearance. Using exercise, specifically aerobic walking, inches are lost faster than weight; and so the tape measure will be more truthful than the scale.

Changes in specific physical features also indicate improvement, such as a less prominent double chin or a hollow developing under each cheekbone.

Another way to measure progress is by your dress or suit size. It is a convenient sum of all your measurements.

The final say on size goes to David A. Rives, author of *Walk Yourself Thin,* who suggests a new unit of measure called the *size-pound,* which he defines as the amount of space that a pound of fat takes up. A pound of muscle takes up more space than a pound of bone, and a pound of fat, still more. Fat is the principal agent of size.

Body fat has not always been a curse. It has not always been a just reprisal for the pleasures of eating or for nature's bountiful offering of the cocoa bean. As *Homo sapiens* evolved, metabolic provision was made for those times when there was less food available than required for the energy needs of daily activity. Those individuals who were able to store extra calories in the form of fat survived when plant and animal food was scarce, and they passed that metabolic trait on to their descendants, us. Now we must learn how to live with a hereditary caloric efficiency that we no longer need.

It is important to remember that our bodies require a little fat in different forms for several vital structures and functions: Sebaceous glands keep the skin supple and the hair luxuriant; nerve sheaths allow effective nerve impulse transmission; fat is a component of mother's milk, a molecular component of several hormones, and a vehicle for the fat-soluble vitamins. You can take care of the essentials with a relatively low-fat diet if the fat is varied and of good quality.

The total amount of fat in the body, including both vital-function lipids and fat stored in fat cells, need be only a small percentage of total body weight. Athletes and dancers can look great and remain healthy at approximately 10 percent fat in males and 20 percent fat in females. Some studies have measured male dancers as low as 7 percent fat and female dancers down to 17 percent. Elite marathoners may be around 5 percent. But you need not be so strict with yourself. At close to 10 percent or 20 percent, male or female respectively, you would look unquestionably lean and yet not risk injury or illness.

Several investigations have shown that exercise walking can lower body fat percentages. One study, reported by Michael M. Pollock and his coworkers at Wake Forest College, was done with 40- to 56-year-old men. Over a period of 20 weeks the experimental subjects walked just over three miles, four times a week, at a little faster than 13 minutes per mile. Compared to the control group who did not exercise, they reduced weight, fat as a percentage of body weight, and skinfold measurements of fat. Another study, reported by Mary M. Cowan and Larry W. Gregory at Western New Mexico University, examined a group of women between the ages of 35 of 66. The experimental group walked four times a week for nine weeks, gradually increasing workout time from 17 minutes to 44 minutes at a target heart rate of 60 percent of maximal. At the end of the nine weeks the subjects in the exercise group had significantly lowered their percentage of body fat whereas those in the control group had not.

In both studies, the actual changes were not large. Both the men and women showed an average of one percent less body fat after these experimental programs. The subjects were not instructed in walking technique, and the only guidance they received was to use heart rate as a measure of intensity. Had they used proper aerobic walking technique, the larger muscle mass used for power would have created greater metabolic change and greater fat loss.

In addition to being undesirable as too high a percentage of total body weight, fat has a bad name for causing the uneven skin surfaces called *cellulite*. Cellulite is not some renegade type of fat. Rather, the nature of animal fat cells is such that they can enlarge and store more and more fat. The connective tissue fibers between groups of fat cells do not stretch to an equal extent, and so we get the typical bulges and dimples. The antidote is aerobic walking which works in two ways to eliminate the cellulite: First, it changes fat-to-lean ratios by reducing the overall amount of stored fat in the body. That flattens the bulges fast. Significant fat reduction takes place within a few weeks. Second, aerobic training increases the elasticity of the connective tissues and so smooths out the cellulite dimples.

Shape

Weight and size respond well to dietary restriction. Shape does not. An individual can diet with a vengeance and become thin. Fat will be lost, but a protruding belly will not be flattened. Muscles of the arms and especially the legs will be ribbon-like rather than spindle shaped, and bones will not become stronger. The weight lost from dieting is not only in fat but also in water and lean tissue.

Aerobic walking, in contrast to only dieting, yields a slim figure with only fat loss. There is a slight gain in lean tissue, and the cells of the vital tissues and organs are better able to utilize water in their metabolism. The muscles used in the exercise become toned and shaped, and—with no fat to hide them—their beautiful long curves show.

Aerobic walking provides strong primary exercise for the hamstring and gluteal muscle groups. In profile, the hamstring tendons show cleanly, and the curve of the hamstring muscles gives the back of the thigh a lean bow shape. Shaping also occurs in the gluteal muscle groups, resulting in a smaller, more rounded fanny.

Aerobic walking requires some modest work from the abdominal muscles. It is not as demanding of these muscles as doing sit-ups, but it is sustained for a longer time. Aerobic walking helps to flatten the tummy by burning fat and by toning the abdominal muscles.

When one puts on weight, the location is determined by heredity, individual chemistry, and sex.

Men tend to store their extra weight in their midsection. We have all seen obese men whose legs and butts are relatively normal in size. The weight in these men is concentrated around the abdomen. They may have waist sizes that measure 45 inches or more with hips that are not at all oversized.

Women are more likely to add weight on their thighs and hips. There are women who are narrow-waisted with sleek upper torsos who have larger legs and posteriors. Rochelle is a friend who is slim and shapely above the waist. Below, she is sizes larger. Despite dieting and playing fierce hours of tennis, she cannot equalize the disparate halves of her body.

Research has identified some of the metabolic gremlins that place fat on the trunk of one individual and on the hips of the next. The gender differences were well noted by the investigators who found strong familial tendencies to gain weight. Other studies concluded that men who exercise aerobically lose more subcutaneous fat on the abdomen than elsewhere on the body. Easy on, easy off.

Females on low-calorie diets did not reduce fat more easily in any particular area. But researchers have found that women who exercise aerobically improve insulin, triglyceride, and total cholesterol levels, all of which are known to increase and decrease in tandem with abdominal fat storage. A similar study of women who exercised aerobically tested their fat cells for responsiveness to adrenalin. The findings showed that subcutaneous abdominal fat was more easily metabolized than was lower body fat. Although we may not conclude definitively that women who exercise will reduce abdominal fat more easily than fat located elsewhere, the evidence is strongly suggestive.

My own clinical observation of both men and women in walking programs is that those who tend to put on weight around their middle will shrink their waistlines with aerobic walking within a few weeks. Fat in other areas of the body comes off according to the dictates of heredity and the individual's metabolism. The bottom line is that your body will make some serious size and shape changes if you are serious about your workouts.

Everyone has a personal notion of what it means to be thin, slim, lean, sleek, and so on. Lean can mean little fat, thin muscles, and lightweight bones. Lean can also mean little fat and strong muscles and bones. If you choose the latter definition, aerobic walking is the path for you.

Posture

Posture is an important part of the total esthetic picture you present. Proud posture adds to the illusion of height and self-assurance, important facets of attractiveness.

Aerobic walking provides mild, sustained exercise for the lower back muscles in balance with the abdominal muscles. It is wonderful for posture. Aerobic walking form also requires the head to be held high and in line with the body's center of gravity, a further contribution to posture. A more detailed analysis of proper aerobic walking form will be presented in chapter 3.

Grace

Shape and posture represent the three-dimensional facets of the esthetics of our bodies. A great shape is shown to best advantage by good posture, but posture can be taken a step further—into the fourth dimension of movement. The smoothness of stride and the strength, yet seeming ease, of movement adds life to posture.

Recently, the columnist Jimmy Breslin interviewed Patricia Donnelly, Miss America of 1939. She recalled, "I had good legs, but the walk was what won for me." Breslin noted that even now she "walked with that smooth winner's stride . . . a straight, firm, even walk that took over the room and caused you to see nothing else."

We in the industrialized world must have lessons in graceful movement. The conveniences of modern civilization have made us into sitters instead of walkers. In a number of low-tech regions around the world, women carry large loads on their heads—no hands—striding easily and smoothly over unpaved ground. Their heads and bodies do not bob up and down as they walk, and the head-borne burdens stay balanced. They walk so smoothly that if you watched only the head and shoulders of such a woman, you would think she was gliding on roller skates.

We, in contrast, walk with a stride that initially decelerates, then accelerates, at every footfall. Our style of walking has been described as falling forward and catching ourselves as each heel comes in contact with the ground. The tops of our heads move up and down, and the overall motion of our bodies is more sporadic than fluid.

Aerobic walking technique is close to that of the native women described above. It is smooth with a light heel strike. The fluid motion of aerobic walking spares the knees and spine from any jarring, enabling even runners with chronic knee problems to obtain a good workout. The smooth stride-to-stride transition can be learned by anyone.

Jean Dalrymple is a good example. She first took up aerobic walking at age 89. After eight lessons she became very smooth and, for her age, swift. She told me that one of her friends had commented on her walking ability: "Jean, you don't walk; you float." Jean is telling us just by her walking that there is no age limit on grace.

Presence

Presence comes from a combination of posture, stride, self-confidence, energy, and a certain *je ne sais quoi*. Aerobic walking does not automatically confer presence. Aerobic walking will, however, bring you the elements that contribute to that special essence.

As you become adept at the technique of aerobic walking and work out at levels that bring metabolic change, you can expect:

o A slimmer, stronger body

o Tall, proud posture

o Movement that is both purposeful and effortless

o Vitality

o Enhanced self-esteem

Finally, esthetics must take into account the qualities of youth. Looking younger is a part of looking good. Aerobic walking, by granting vitality and a strong stride, will bestow a more youthful appearance. Healthy, beautiful, and young! What could be better?

CHAPTER 2

Metabolic Magic
How to Become a Lean Machine

Dale is one of my brightest friends. She is logical in her thinking and knowledgeable on a broad range of subjects, including the sciences. Yet, Dale says, "I don't care what the doctors and nutritionists say about calories and pounds; I just look at food and get fat."

Dale, of course, is using the words "look at food" as a metaphor for how sparingly she eats. Recent studies have proven her to be right. Different people process food in different ways—some more efficiently, some less so. Metabolism does differ from one person to another, and even in the same person metabolism will respond to changes in eating habits and exercise.

Metabolism—Play, Reverse, and Fast Forward

Everyone's energy equation equals the sum of the following pluses and minuses:

+ The caloric content of diet
+ How many of those calories are absorbed from the gastrointestinal tract
− The calories expended to digest, absorb, and use the nutrients from the diet
− The caloric cost of all other basic functions of the body such as breathing, thinking, growing, secreting, excreting, and healing
− The caloric cost of more active musculoskeletal work in daily activities and exercise

Each of these energy pluses and minuses is handled differently in different people. The complaints of those who find it easy to gain and difficult to lose weight ought not be taken lightly. Metabolic rates are influenced by several factors. Some are under the individual's control; some are not. The factors include:

1. Heredity

2. Diet

3. Exercise

4. Gender

5. Endocrine activity

6. Age

This chapter provides some insight into the body's metabolic ways, especially the relationship between exercise and diet. Exercise is important in losing weight and critical to the maintenance of weight loss.

Heredity

In 1990, Claude Bouchard and his team of investigators at Laval University in Quebec reported their study of pairs of twins, which sought to determine the hereditability of weight gain. In an overfeeding experiment, the scientists found little variation in regional fat distribution and the amount of intra-abdominal fat between any two twins of a pair and great variation from one pair to another. There was six times as much variance among pairs as within pairs. Other measures—body weight, percentage of fat, and total fat—showed three times as much variance among pairs as within pairs.

Albert Stunkard and a team at the University of Pennsylvania, in another twins study reported that same year, collected data on height and weight in pairs who had been reared together and pairs who had been reared apart. Stunkard compared similarities and differences in body mass index (weight in kilograms divided by the square of height in meters). He found that among all the factors influencing body mass, genetic influences had the strongest determining role. The genetic influence on weight gain was more than twice as important as personal and situational influences such as food preferences and luncheon meetings at work.

Heredity also influences our levels of exercise and physical activity. Those who blame their genes for their tight jeans seem to have a valid argument. Heredity, however, is not enough reason to give up and be fat. Dr. Stunkard says, "Hereditability [of body mass] does not imply an invariant, immutable genetic influence such as occurs in the case of hair or eye color." Heredity is only an influence and only one influence at that. Other influences, particularly diet and exercise, can be used to override the metabolic commands of an unfavorable inheritance. Knowing how your metabolism responds to less or more food and less or more exercise will provide you with valuable information. Put this knowledge to work for you.

Diet

Let us first look at the basic facts about calories and metabolism.

o We need about 500 calories per day for fundamentals such as breathing, eating, and just sitting around.

o In sedentary adults, 75 percent of total caloric expenditure is accounted for by the body's metabolic processes.

o Those who exercise burn many more calories than their sedentary counterparts, with only 5 percent to 10 percent of total calories expended on resting metabolism.

Restrictive dieting influences not only weight and size, it can change the body's metabolism and make it easy to gain the weight back. Ninety-nine percent of all people who want to lose weight go on some sort of a diet. It is their perception that if they eat less they will lose more. If the equation *eating less = losing more* were a physical law, losing weight would be a straightforward matter. But we are dealing with biology, not physics, in the science of reducing, and we must understand biology's wry sense of humor to be successful in losing weight and not regaining it.

Food and Nutrients. Different bodies handle proteins, carbohydrates, and fats in different ways. An exercise-trained body and a sedentary body may handle these nutrients somewhat differently, but there are common denominators as well. Each of the nutrients deserves to be examined in some detail.

Proteins: Dietary protein is vital in both normal and weight-loss diets. Protein supplies the amino acids that are the building blocks of cells, tissues, and vital organs. Protein is the sole source of ten essential amino acids that the human body cannot manufacture from raw materials. All ten—arginine, histidine, isoleucine, leucine, lysine, methionine, phenylalanine, threonine, tryptophan, and valine—are present in proteins from animal sources and in proteins from pairs of vegetable sources. There are other amino acids used in protein metabolism that the body *can* assemble from its molecular inventory. Both types of amino acids are necessary for the regeneration, repair, and maintenance of the tissues of the body.

Some of the essential amino acids are used in metabolically specific ways to keep the body functioning well. For example:

o Tryptophan is the precursor of serotonin which, in turn, regulates appetite and sexual function and helps to block mental depression.

o Methionine contributes to the formation of acetyl choline, a neurotransmitter used for the transmission of most nerve impulses, including those to the muscles used in workouts.

o Phenylalanine takes part in the formation of adrenalin and thyroid hormone.

o Arginine and histadine are important for growth in children and needed at all ages for proper liver and kidney function.

o Isoleucine, leucine, and valine can be used as a supplementary energy resource in exercise.

There is a constant tissue turnover in our bodies, requiring dietary protein for replacement on a regular basis. Exercise increases the protein needs of the body, depending on the intensity and duration of the workout. Weight-loss diets can cause protein breakdown and loss. You should not lose weight at the expense of protein in the cells of muscle, bone, and vital organs. You need protein as you become lean.

Carbohydrates: When you eat carbohydrates (sugars and starches), your body has choices of what to do with them. They can be used in any combination of the following three ways:

1. Carbohydrates can go into the blood as glucose to be used for energy needs.
2. Carbohydrates can be stored in the liver and muscles as glycogen.
3. Carbohydrates can be converted into fat.

Simple sugars—such as syrups or table sugar—are absorbed quickly from the intestinal tract and, in large part, must be released into the systemic blood stream, often in larger amounts than the body can use at one time. The body responds by releasing insulin, which causes an increased metabolic breakdown of glucose and a fall in blood sugar. Starches—such as breads, rice, and potatoes—are digested and absorbed more slowly and can be utilized and stored in more deliberate ways.

A body that is exercise-trained has many advantages over a sedentary body in the metabolic arena of using and storing carbohydrates. A trained body can better utilize carbohydrates because it has greater numbers of and more sensitive insulin receptors in the cells of the body's tissues. Insulin stimulates these receptors to metabolize excess blood glucose. A trained body also has a greater capacity to store carbohydrate as glycogen in liver and muscle tissues, further stabilizing blood sugar levels. These metabolic improvements result in less carbohydrate being stored as fat.

Blood sugar levels are very sensitive to what you eat and how well your body handles carbohydrates. The reason is plain to see when you look at the simple mathematics involved. Suppose you were to eat a generous piece of pecan pie. Except for the pecans, eggs, and butter, it is mostly corn syrup and brown sugar. Let's suppose a slice of pecan pie provides 600 calories of which 400 calories are derived from simple sugar. That estimate is probably close to accurate. The 400 calories equal 100 grams of carbohydrate (1 gram of carbohydrates = 4 calories). So much for the mathematics of the *pie* (Figure 1).

Now let's see about *blood sugar*. Normal blood sugar is about 100 milligrams of glucose per 100 cc of blood. The total blood vol-

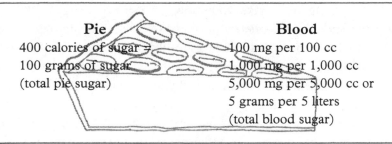

Pie	Blood
400 calories of sugar =	100 mg per 100 cc
100 grams of sugar	1,000 mg per 1,000 cc
(total pie sugar)	5,000 mg per 5,000 cc or
	5 grams per 5 liters
	(total blood sugar)

Figure 1. In a slice of pecan pie, the amount of carbohydrate in the form of simple sugar is twenty times the body's total blood sugar. Counsel: Eat slowly and don't even think about doubles.

ume of the average person is about 5 liters (a little over 5 quarts); 100 mg of glucose per 100 cc of blood is equal to 1,000 mg (1 gram) of glucose per 1,000 cc (1 liter) of blood or 5 grams of glucose in 5 liters.

It is a stark comparison: Total blood glucose is 5 grams. Total glucose in one slice of pie is *100* grams!

If the body did not have various mechanisms of using, diverting, and storing the sugar, the blood stream would be its destination. The pie's 100 grams of sugar—20 times the amount of sugar in the entire blood stream—would drive the blood sugar to 2,000 mg per 100 cc. That would produce diabetic coma two or three times over!

We obviously do not go into diabetic coma every time we eat a sugary dessert. How do we manage the oversupply? The blood sugar does rise, but it generally stays well below 200. The liver does not allow too much of the sugar to enter the blood stream at once; the pancreas produces more insulin; the liver and muscles convert some of the glucose into glycogen; the liver converts some into fat; and there are other mechanisms as well.

We can appreciate the slim margin of safety within which the body works to keep blood sugar close to the 100 mg level. This example points up the need to maintain an optimal state of health to handle such emergencies as a slice of pecan pie.

Dietary Fats: An exercise-trained body is better than a sedentary body in dealing with dietary fat. Training will reduce the production of triglycerides, one of the bad guys in the blood lipid profile. Training will make you more efficient at using circulating free fatty acids for the energy needs of exercise. Physiological measurements have shown an increasing utilization of free fatty acids by the working muscles through 75 minutes of an aerobic workout. If your diet is modest in fat content and you exercise regularly, you will likely use up all the fat in your diet and have none left to store in all the familiar places. Exercise can overcome an occasional small portion of a delicious dessert; and that occasional taste delight will keep you from feeling totally deprived.

A proviso: Exercise can do wondrous things, but it cannot undo the effects of high-fat foods if they are a regular part of your diet. High fat content in food is a disaster for dieters in at least two ways.

First, fat is rich in calories. One gram of fat contains nine calories, versus four calories per gram of carbohydrates and four calories per gram of protein. Nine calories doesn't sound like much, but a gram isn't much either. Translated to ounces, there are over 200 calories per ounce of fat!

Second, after dietary fat is digested, the body can easily convert it back into fat for deposit in the fat cells of the body. A diet with excess fat calories will increase weight and percentage of body fat faster than a diet with excess carbohydrate or protein calories.

Reducing Diets. Reducing diets are always low in something—protein, fat, carbohydrates, calories, or taste. All of these diets influence metabolism. And, of course, less food provides less nutrition.

Low Carbohydrate Diets: Low carbohydrate diets, even to the point of no carbohydrates at all, work well for losing weight. Too few carbohydrates is not a good idea.

The sedentary body needs about 500 calories just for basic metabolism and minimal activity. Dietary carbohydrate, because it is directly converted to glucose and glycogen, is the body's preferred energy source. Without this minimum 500 calories in carbohydrates, the body will convert fat and, to a lesser extent, protein to glucose for energy needs. In the process, organic acids called *ketones* are produced. These acids depress cellular function in a wide spectrum of tissues, including the brain. The centers of the brain that control appetite and mood are especially affected. Thus, ketosis is a double-edged sword—appetite becomes depressed but so do your spirits.

Outside the brain, the organic acids decrease pH (acidity) of both blood and tissue fluids, upseting the balance of potassium between the tissue fluids and the cells. This electrolyte disturbance can affect muscle contraction and even diminish normal heart activity. Endocrine balance, kidney function, bone metabolism, and many of the other functions of the body are also thrown into disarray.

Very Low-Calorie Diets (under 500 calories and under medical supervision): Very low-calorie diets, as well as low carbohydrate diets, are associated with ketosis and the suppression of cellular function. A further disadvantage of very low-calorie diets is that metabolic rate is sharply reduced. Several studies have shown that the rate decreases by 13 percent to 24 percent below pre diet levels. With this metabolic slowdown, it becomes more difficult to continue losing weight. Resistance and plateaus result, and it becomes a struggle to reach your goal weight. If you finally do reach your goal and change from a weight-loss diet to a maintenance diet, there will be other metabolic gremlins waiting.

First, your metabolic rate, which slowed down on the restricted diet, does not quite return to prediet levels, making your body metabolically worse off than if there had been no dieting at all.

Second, fat deposition can increase with each meal. The chemical culprit is an enzyme called *lipoprotein lipase*. Found in fatty tissues, lipoprotein lipase acts to increase the synthesis of fat for tissue storage. While weight is actively being lost, lipoprotein lipase is at low levels. After starting on a maintenance diet, lipoprotein lipase increases sharply following digestion.

Third, after losing weight, ketone-induced unhappiness may lead you to seek the solace of "real food" to make up for the weeks of deprivation. The solace food is often eaten in such quantities and at such a rate that mealtime becomes a feeding frenzy.

The overall result is the regaining of all the lost weight, plus a few pounds, often in less time than it took to lose it. Be careful with very low-calorie diets.

Low-Fat Diets: Every body needs a certain amount of fat (lipid) for normal functioning.

o Many nerves have protective sheaths which, in good part, are made up of lipids. An example is the white matter of the brain.

o Prostaglandins, the on-site group of hormone-like substances found in many of the tissues of the body, rely on lipids to supply key components of their molecular structure.

o Free fatty acids of the blood can be drawn upon as an energy source for skeletal muscle contraction.

o HDL (high density lipoprotein), the coronary protective factor that counters the harmful effects of LDL (low density lipoprotein), is lipid-based.

For much of this metabolic chemistry, the body uses essential fatty acids which, like the essential amino acids, cannot be manufactured "in house." Dietary fat is their only source.

How do you make sure you are meeting these vital needs? Do not worry. It is almost impossible to reduce the fat content of your diet to dangerously low levels. A diet in which only ten percent of total calories are fat can supply all the essentials. A diet that is only ten percent fat is so plain tasting, no one would, by choice or chance, forego every last fat-containing treat just to stay within the diet guidelines. A low-fat diet that is varied and healthful will also supply the fat-based vitamins A, D, E, and K. A low-fat diet can bring about weight loss without any of the doubts or dangers of some of the other types of diets. I recommend it as a complement to aerobic walking for weight loss.

Exercise for Metabolic Magic

Losing weight on a diet involves losing fat, water, and lean tissue. The loss of lean tissue is one of the reasons for the slowing of metabolic rate in very low-calorie diets. Lean tissue is the dominant force on the metabolic fast track; losing lean tissue means less force-driving metabolism. Fat cells contribute proportionally little to overall metabolic rate.

When aerobic exercise is added to a calorically restricted diet, three positive things happen:

First, the slowed metabolic rate speeds up to prediet levels (Figure 2).

Second, the amount of fat loss increases dramatically, more than doubling the loss from diet alone (Figure 3). Remember that fat is the strongest determinant of size.

Third, the lean tissue loss is reversed, actually increasing slightly above prediet values (Figure 3). An exercise-induced increase in lean tissue will create a healthy feeling, and your muscles will become firm and well shaped.

Exercise can also increase energy output in three major ways.

First, the differences between the total calories burned by sedentary individuals and the calories burned by those who exercise regularly can be enormous. In sedentary individuals, resting metabolism accounts for 75 percent of total caloric expenditure. In exercising individuals, only 10 percent of total caloric expenditure is from resting metabolism. The rest (90 percent) is from the work the muscles are delivering. That is the first advantage of exercise—direct, substantial burning of calories.

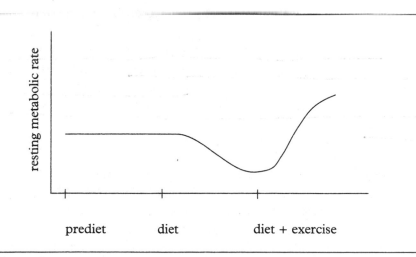

Figure 2.

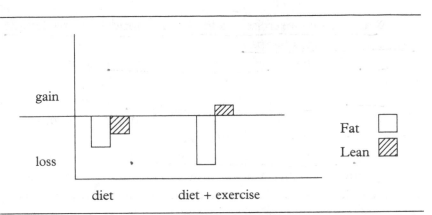

Figure 3.

Second, those who exercise regularly increase the thermic effect of digestion, which means an increased use of calories in digesting their meals.

Third, even after the workout is over there is an afterburn. Metabolic rate naturally rises during exercise. When exercise stops, the metabolic rate *gradually* returns to pre-exercise levels. The time for that gradual return may be as little as a few minutes or as long as 24 to 48 hours, depending on the workout. A long, strong workout using large muscle groups yields a longer, higher residual metabolic rate. The higher post-exercise rate will remain above resting levels even as you are resting.

Exercise is the only way, other than drugs, to change your metabolism to that of a naturally slim person. The cost-benefit ratio would delight an accountant—a 45-*minute* workout yields 24 or more *hours* of a metabolism that you might otherwise sell your soul for.

No Pain, No Gain? "No pain, no gain" is the mirror image of the philosophy that says of food, "If it tastes so good, it can't be healthy." In the realm of food, that philosophy is often correct. Many of the great tasting foods are less than healthful, and invariably they are fattening. The philosophy doesn't hold for exercise. Physical pain does not guarantee an aerobic effect. Physical effort and the mental tenacity to exert that effort for the entire workout don't have to hurt.

If you feel pain during the workout, it is a message from some part of your body either to slow down or to adjust your form. Chest pain, because it may be a sign of an acute cardiac problem, is a signal to stop and seek help immediately. Musculoskeletal pain is addressed in chapter 9, "Safely, Safely."

Sometimes you will feel impatient for the workout to be over. Sometimes you will not feel like doing a workout at all. Sometimes you won't like the feeling of being a little out of breath for 45 minutes. You will be able, with a little concentration, to work through these psychological discomforts.

Exercise and Brain Chemistry. The brain is a chemical plant as much as it is a computerized switchboard. There are over 30 neurotransmitter chemicals—norepinephrine, serotonin, and dopamine are three of the principal ones—that are produced in the various parts of the brain and which, in health, are in balance through their daily cycles. When in balance they will:

o Keep appetite in line with caloric needs
o Promote emotional stability
o Support self-esteem
o Maintain mental energy at a high level
o Prevent mild to moderate mental depression
o Enable you to react well to stressful situations

All of these effects are important in losing weight. They are even more important for maintaining the new weight permanently. These desirable effects are not merely psychological in origin; they are the result of actual changes in brain chemistry. As such they are primary metabolic improvements that will bring permanent slimness.

Upgrading Exercise. The metabolic changes that result from exercise occur principally in the working muscles at the muscle cell level. The more muscle cells (or total muscle mass) enlisted in the exercise, the greater the amount of metabolic change. Small muscles produce small metabolic change, and large muscles produce large metabolic change.

To gain maximum benefit, choose an exercise and an exercise technique that use large muscle groups, preferably several of them. The muscles must be used in a continuous, rhythmic, repetitive fashion. Thresholds of distance, intensity, and frequency (how far, how fast, how often) must also be met.

Aerobic walking fits all the criteria of a high-grade aerobic exercise. No wonder it is so effective for weight-loss programs. You will see and feel the resultant changes in your metabolism in only a few weeks.

Aerobic walking also has other advantages: It is safe, convenient, inexpensive, suitable for all ages, and requires no special equipment or facilities. It is the best exercise for all seasons and for all reasons.

Many charts have been devised to show how many calories different exercises consume. There are charts for calories per hour and per mile, calories per hour at different speeds, and minutes to burn up a four-ounce hamburger. The charts generally rate walking at 2, 3, and 4 mph. Occasionally a chart lists walking at 5 mph. The chart in figure 4 gives a basic guide for calories burned during the exercise period using ordinary brisk walking. Aerobic walking, which uses the largest muscle groups of the lower body, would consume many more calories and then keep your metabolic rate high for a longer time after your workout. This chart is a general guide for average-sized people—not very large and not very small.

Know Your Body's Limits. Many people on diets are impatient with their progress and are willing to be extremist for a while to get faster results. Exercise at optimal aerobic levels can keep you in the pink while you are losing weight and size. Exercise that is excessive can lead to physiological and musculoskeletal blues.

Pace	Calories Per Mile	
	Average Female	Average Male
3 mph	50 to 80	80 to 100
4 mph	60 to 90	90 to 110
5 mph	70 to 110	105 to 125

Figure 4. The number of calories you will burn depends on your weight, your walking style, and your pace.

Overtraining can result in muscle, joint, and/or tendon trauma. Even stress fractures can occur. Almost all competitive athletes, especially at world-class levels, train beyond the needs of health. Many of them suffer severe injuries, sometimes requiring surgery. But this level of training is far more than the three hours or so per week that you will do.

Exercise, done right, has a powerful impact. It can counter the effects of a disadvantaged heredity. It can reverse the effects of many disease states. It can neutralize two or three thousand extra calories per week in a diet.

Exercise can do some miraculous things at less-than-extreme levels of time and effort. Chapters 3 and 4 provide guidance on technique and thresholds of how far, how fast, and how often.

Gender

Women and men are different—anatomically and hormonally. Taking the cardiovascular system as one example, women have substantial protection from heart attacks until menopause. Their estrogen levels provide this immunity, although it is not an absolute guarantee for all women under all conditions. After menopause, this natural immunity is lost, and then some. Of all patients who suffer heart attacks, fewer women than men survive the acute phase, and more women than men are struck with a second attack within a year.

As another example, women have a higher percentage of body fat than men. Fat cells contribute far less to the body's metabolic rate than lean tissue cells do. Men, having a higher percentage of muscle tissues, naturally have a higher metabolic rate. Thus, a woman could gain weight and a man could lose weight on the very same diet. Even when exercising at aerobic levels, women still have to be prudent about their diets. "Prudent" does not mean deprived, but merely going easy on fats and calories.

A Canadian study by Bhambhani and Singh at the University of Alberta correlated some of the influences on exercise metabolism: running versus walking, men versus women, and exercise technique. The investigators found that there was no difference between the sexes in the metabolic cost of walking, but that the metabolic cost of running was significantly higher in women.

In teaching aerobic walking I have found that women generally pick up the form more easily and are able to increase their speed dramatically.

Despite the physical differences between the sexes, men and women can both excel at walking.

Endocrine Activity

Gender, as we all know, is controlled by a balance of the sex hormones—estrogen (female) and testosterone (male). The sex hormones, while they are at it, influence muscle mass and fat storage. Men, under the influence of testosterone, can build up the size, shape, and strength of their muscles with weight lifting or other resistance exercises. Women, having only minimal testosterone levels, can increase strength but cannot produce the muscle size that men can.

The body's metabolism and the tendency toward weight/size gain is also influenced by other hormones such as thyroid hormone, insulin, adrenalin, and the adrenal steroids. Thyroid hormone can increase metabolic rates and heart rate. Insulin increases the rate of glucose utilization. Adrenalin and cortisone influence fat and carbohydrate metabolism. Hormone synthesis and function, in turn, are influenced by all the other factors that contribute to the metabolic bottom line: heredity, diet, exercise, gender, and age. Diet and exercise are the two that you have control over. Diet and exercise give you a strong say in your own metabolism.

Age

When I was a small boy growing up in Brooklyn, my grandparents' apartment in Williamsburg was the family meeting place. I remember discussions among my grandfather, my father, and two or three uncles on the subjects of business and health. Politics was not discussed much. It was wartime, and patriotism and general unity were not to be questioned.

When health was discussed, the issue of blood pressure always came up. Both my maternal grandparents were hypertensive, and at that time a low-salt diet was the only treatment. The consensus was that normal blood pressure should be figured at 100 plus one's age. Systolic pressure was the all-important figure. My grandfather's pressure of 170, therefore, was not alarming for his age of 68.

That generation believed that other inexorable changes accompanied advancing years. Memory was not as sharp, physical strength declined, and both mental and physical agility were reduced. When you got old, you got old. It was an accepted premise.

Since World War II, an ever-increasing amount of research has been done in the field of sports and exercise. The initial work concentrated on athletes and their physiology as compared to a sedentary population. As the results of the many studies—both laboratory and field work—were collected, there emerged a general pattern of beneficial health changes following endurance training. It was not long before some investigators decided to find out about older athletes and then older sedentary people who underwent exercise training.

The wealth of knowledge that has been collected in the postwar period has challenged the tenets of my grandparents' and parents' generations. No longer are "hardening of the arteries" and a systolic blood pressure of 100 plus age necessary consequences of senior citizenship. It is now accepted that more than half the decline of aging is attributable to inactivity, not chronological years.

Many studies have shown that exercise can bring about strong improvement in almost all the metabolic functions that ordinarily decline with increasing years. There does not seem to be any age limit for this reversal of the effects of inactivity.

In a multicenter study, Maria A. Fiatarone and her coworkers observed a group of nonagenarians who were given resistance training for eight weeks. The oldsters showed strength gains averaging 174 percent over pretraining levels! The men and the women in the study made equally dramatic gains.

In other studies, seniors in exercise programs experienced gains in quickness of thinking, increases in maximal oxygen power, lowering of hypertensive blood pressures, and other improvements in metabolic function.

Change also occurs with not-so-advanced age. A survey of weight changes at various ages concluded that the most significant weight gain in the general population occurs in the 25 to 34 age range. It is the very age that coincides with the change from active college days to a life of employment with its more sedentary lifestyle. Inactivity must be counted as a prime suspect as the cause of obesity in the under 35 age category.

Metabolism may be awesomely, dauntingly complicated. It may be controlled in good measure by your parents and grandparents. All is not lost, though. You can influence your metabolism by means of diet and exercise. These two factors together can help to keep your metabolism in balance.

CHAPTER 3

Aerobic Walking
Technique Is Everything

An old friend, who is world renowned as a poet/philosopher knows that I teach aerobic walking as a preventive medicine and weight-loss exercise. He laughs at the concept.

"Why don't you teach people how to sit or stand or swallow their food?" he chides me.

Others, too, have made fun of the concept of learning how to walk after age two.

Studies have been done to determine how effective walking is as an exercise. The results varied with the age, sex, and fitness levels of the subjects. Old and less-fit individuals made moderate gains in aerobic power (measured as maximal oxygen capacity). Subjects in their 20s and 30s and those who were highly fit did *not* improve their levels of fitness unless they reached a speed of 5 mph (12 minutes per mile) in their workouts. The studies reported that the subjects found it biomechanically difficult to walk at such a pace (Duncan; Porcari).

To underscore the importance of pace in exercise walking, John J. Duncan and his coworkers at the Cooper Institute for Aerobic Research reported a 24-week study that measured oxygen power in women before and after three differently-paced walking programs. The investigators found that strolling, brisk walking, and aerobic-pace walking produced, respectively, mild, moderate, and strong increases in fitness. In all cases the distance was the same. The aerobic-pace walking, in fact, was found to be as effective as jogging for improving fitness.

I personally have seen how difficult it is for individuals to shift their walking speed into high gear on their own. In the aerobic walking

29

program at the New Age Health Spa, I have been testing participants as they enter the program by using a chart of age-graded fitness levels in conjunction with a timed, one-mile walk (Figure 5).
Among 50 individuals tested thus far, only two have exceeded a pace
of 5 mph. One was a 28-year-old male who is an active runner. The
other was a 35-year-old woman who had previously taken classes in
aerobic walking technique.

One-Mile Walk Fitness Test

Age	Low Fitness	Moderate Fitness	High Fitness
20 to 30	over 16 minutes	11.5 to 16 minutes	under 11.5 minutes
30 to 40	over 17 minutes	12 to 17 minutes	under 12 minutes
40 to 50	over 18 minutes	13 to 18 minutes	under 13 minutes
50 to 60	over 19 minutes	13.5 to 19 minutes	under 13.5 minutes
60 to 70	over 20 minutes	14 to 20 minutes	under 14 minutes
over 70	over 22 minutes	15 to 22 minutes	under 15 minutes

Figure 5.

All the work in the laboratories and in the field seems to be saying that walking has its limits and is, at best, a modest aerobic exercise.
Yet, I propose that aerobic walking is an exercise equal to cross-country
skiing in effectiveness. Whom can you believe? Can both be right?

Actually, both are correct; we are talking about different kinds
of walking. *Ordinary brisk walking* is not a high-grade exercise for
producing metabolic change in your body. But *aerobic walking* is a
remarkably effective exercise for bringing about beneficial health
and esthetic changes.

Increasing Your Walking Speed

Anatomy and Mechanics

If walking is such a simple skill that everyone uses it everyday
without a second thought, why is it so difficult to walk faster than 5
mph? One reason that has been advanced is that as walking speed

approaches 5 mph it becomes easier to run. That is true, but it does not address the biomechanics of the question.

Analyzing Gait. An analysis of gait anatomy and mechanics shows that:

1. In ordinary brisk walking, the calf muscles are the principal source of power.
2. In ordinary brisk walking, each foot is placed on the ground in a distinctly separate step—left, right, left, right—which makes it difficult to increase stride rate (steps per minute).
3. Aerobic walking uses the largest of muscle groups—hamstrings, gluteals, and trunk muscles—for power.
4. Aerobic walking employs an extremely smooth transition from one stride to the next.

The larger muscles used in aerobic walking can move the body faster. The smooth stride turnover produces a continuous application of power. It is as if one footstep flows into the next, allowing for an almost limitless increase in stride rate.

This smooth, continuous cycling of footsteps can be thought of as a slow-motion version of a cartoon character whose feet are whirling around in a blur. A smooth, gliding technique is as important as using the power class of muscles to attain good speed.

If you are fit and healthy to start with, proper technique will enable you to reach a pace of 12 minutes per mile or better through your entire workout. If you are older, ill or out of shape, you may be able to attain a pace of 13 to 15 minutes per mile by the eighth week of your aerobic walking program. Such a pace will be highly aerobic for your individual body.

A dramatic example of the connection between form and speed is illustrated by my neighbors Rebecca and Marty who took up aerobic walking for stress reduction and weight control. Marty, being stronger, had always been a faster walker than Rebecca, but Rebecca quickly picked up the fluid form and easily became the faster of the two. Marty has since improved, but Rebecca is still ahead in both style and speed.

Techniques for Learning

How we walk has become well ingrained over many years. We have long since given little thought to walking style. It will take some self-awareness and some work to attain the form needed for metabolic change. Improvement is often in small increments, and you will need to be patient with your progress. If you persevere, you will make a breakthrough in technique at some point.

Chantal's experience is a perfect example. Although she is slim and athletic, Chantal initially found it difficult to pick up the stride flow. She was angry with herself for not being able to improve quickly at something as elementary as walking. Then, after about six weeks of practice, a light bulb went on in her neuromuscular system. To her surprise and delight, her form and speed increased dramatically. "*Regardez moi!* I'm flying!" Of course, it took some weeks of effort for it to happen, but once she had the technique in her proprioceptive memory, she was able to walk like the wind every time. Months later, she and I were doing a workout at a strong pace, unaware that we were being observed by a couple of walkers who had previously taken one of my courses. They asked Chantal if she was one of my instructors.

Learning by Parts

There are 21 facets of ideal aerobic walking form:

1. Feet parallel
2. Inside edge of each foot falling on same line—feet neither apart nor overlapped
3. No pronation (the foot leans in); no supination (the foot leans out)
4. Optimal stride length, to be achieved mainly by hip advancement
5. Silent heel contact, then progressive increase in acceleration
6. Gliding rather than hiking motion
7. Heel kept on ground as long as possible without extreme stretching

8. Leg brought forward early at end of ground contact phase of stride (before toe-off)

9. Power in stride, especially from vertical leg position to ball of foot push-off

10. Posture tall but relaxed; overall motion in a forward and upward direction

11. Pelvis and chest leading equally

12. Shoulders relaxed

13. Dissociation of upper and lower body—upper relaxed, and lower producing power

14. Arms bent 90 degrees at the elbow

15. Arms allowed to swing, not forced; back swing at least equal to forward swing

16. Horizontal plane of arm swing describes a slight arc, hands moving from the side of body forward toward the mid-chest line

17. Hip advancement in a forward direction with each stride, not a rotary or lateral motion

18. Flexible hip movement, not rigid

19. Unstrained pace

20. Downhill—faster strides, avoid "catching" oneself at each heel strike

21. Uphill—straight posture, not bent at the waist

This list dispels the notion that aerobic walking is the same as brisk walking with an added wrinkle or two. The technique is complex, and each of the 21 facets of form deserves some elaboration. Later in this chapter, under "The Malkin Technique," the facets are presented in detail in their six natural groups: feet, legs, hips, arms, posture, and gliding. But first, it is important to understand how to learn.

If you try to incorporate all 21 components into your walking style at once, you may look and feel like a spider trying to go in eight directions at once. It is better to start with the walking style you already know and make improvements gradually, one or two at a time. As you become comfortable with each change, you can go on to the next.

In the early stages, your walking form may fall apart to such an extent that you feel ready to give up and go back to your old, inefficient, graceless ways. Don't despair—just hang in there. Everyone, athlete or klutz, will improve over a few short weeks. As you become stronger and smoother, you may not notice the small gains from one session to the next. Just look back to the first workout, and you will appreciate how far you've come.

Learning by Wholes

Breaking aerobic walking down into its 21 component parts and then reassembling the parts is one way of learning. Another way is learning by wholes. By looking at the total-form picture you can absorb technique in an intuitive, almost subconscious way. I remember when I was a teenager in the forties, boys would learn how to dance by practicing the box step. Girls learned by feeling the rhythm of the music and watching their friends dance. The boys learned by parts; the girls learned by wholes. You can integrate both methods and become proficient that much faster.

Learning by wholes will be reinforced each time you watch someone who is good at aerobic walking. Even if it is difficult to critique your own style, you will be able to recognize different levels of skill in other walkers. Pick out the best to emulate. You will absorb their style to some extent just by watching.

Many times when a student in an instructional program is not able to absorb any more detail and analysis, I just walk alongside in silence, keeping my own form as ideal as possible. Learning takes place as if by osmosis.

The Malkin Technique
of Aerobic Walking

Aerobic walking is different than the way you have been walking all these years. In ordinary walking, the body's center of gravity (as well as the level of the top of the head) moves up and down with each stride, whereas in aerobic walking the body glides at the same level. Then, too, there are differences in power, speed, and other fundamentals. It will take a few weeks to pick up the basic technique of aerobic walking; you must be patient. The intellect may learn quickly, but the muscles learn more slowly. If you look at the learning process as both challenging and interesting, it will be so. It can even become fun.

The First Step

Start by lacing your walking shoes a little on the loose side. The form of aerobic walking does not need a tight fit around the instep. The power you will use to propel yourself forward is applied in a backward, downward direction, and this force is exerted against the heel counter. Bending at the ball of the foot will be minimal, resulting in very little tendency to lift the heel out of the shoe.

Footwork—Staying on the Right Track

In aerobic walking, as in other exercises and sports, technique and position are, if not everything, pretty important. Starting at ground level, the feet should be close to parallel to each other, with the inside of the right foot on the same line as the inside of the left foot. The feet should not cross over, one in front of the other, nor should they be separated left and right (Figure 6).

The normal postural anatomy of the feet as you stand is very slightly toed out (Figure 7). When you use proper hip motion (explained later in this chapter), your feet will turn in just enough to bring them parallel.

Foot position is not one of the critical factors in learning aerobic walking technique. If your feet toe in or out a bit, it will not destroy the entire form, just as long as you don't walk like a duck with your feet apart or like a pigeon with the toes of one foot pointing at the toes of the other foot.

Consider also where weight is borne with each stride. *Pronation* occurs when the weight of the body falls on the inside edge (the arch side) of the foot. *Supination* describes the position when the weight

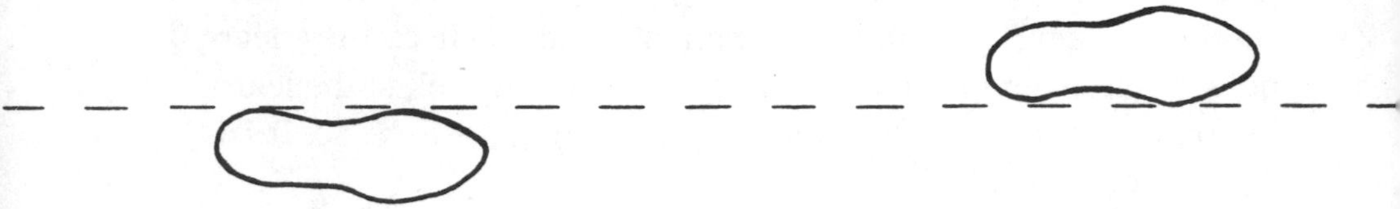

Figure 6.

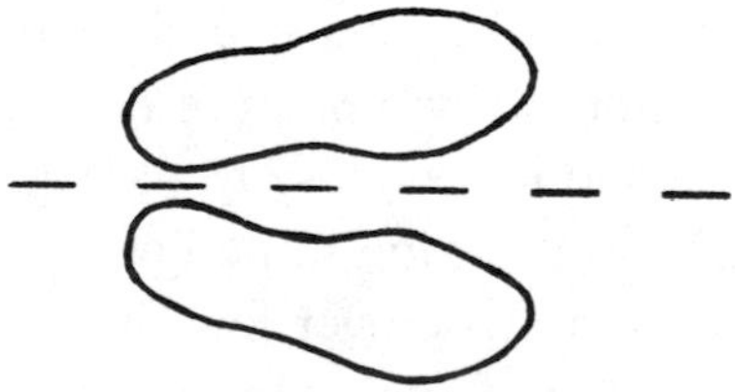

Figure 7.

falls on the outside edge of the support foot. The former is far more common.

Pronation prevents a balanced stride and inhibits a smooth, fast stride turnover. It strains the arch and the ankle, and it places stress on the inner aspect of the knee joint. The wear on the soles of your shoes, especially the heels, tells you if you are pronating. They will look like a tire that is out of alignment with most of the wear on the inner side.

There are three ways to cure pronation. One way is to use an arch support, either a ready-made one sold in shoe shops and pharmacies or a professional one prescribed by a podiatrist. A second way is to use athletic shoes that have a less yielding material on the inside (medial) half of the soles of the shoes. A third way is to concentrate on walking with the pressure of your weight more on the outside half of each foot, which in time becomes a habit. I recommend the third way, which eventually provides stronger ankle support by using your own muscles, tendons, and ligaments.

Getting a Leg up on Power

When you walk, each leg goes through two phases with every stride cycle: the ground (or support) phase and the air (or recovery) phase. In the first, the leg presses the earth backward to move you forward. In the second, the leg is brought forward to be ready for the next stride.

When your heel makes its initial contact with the ground at the very beginning of the ground phase, try to accelerate. That means pulling the earth backward (actually downward and backward) with your heel.

As your heel passes directly under your center of gravity, that leg will be vertical and your entire foot will be touching the ground. Continue pressing the earth backward with the entire foot as if you are rolling a huge log around.

As your foot and leg move backward from the vertical support position, keep the entire foot in contact with the ground as long as you comfortably can. Do not come up on the ball of the foot early; otherwise your whole body will be bopping up and down. As your foot moves behind your center of gravity, increase the strength with which you press the earth backward. Your whole leg will tend to straighten at this point, giving you the feeling that your leg is acting as a giant straight-spring with the fixed point at the hip.

When the ground contact leg has passed so far back that the heel naturally comes off the ground, you will, of course, be on the ball of the foot. At this point, you will automatically push off using the calf muscles to spin the earth a little further backward. You do not need to make an extra effort for this push off. It is already wired into your reflexes.

You will be using the large muscles of the lower body, particularly the hamstring and gluteal groups, to move your leg backward against the resistance of the earth. You need not take my word for it; you can prove it for yourself. As you are standing still, touch the back of your right thigh with your right hand. Then try to move the right foot backward by scraping it on the ground. You will feel the back of the thigh tighten as the hamstring muscles contract. The power for the backward movement of the leg against the resistance of the ground comes particularly from the hamstring group. When you walk with aerobic technique, the action of the hamstrings is the same as what you have just demonstrated for yourself.

Walkers Are "Hip" People

Environmentalists have always thought of walkers as "hip" people. Until now they didn't know it was a literal as well as political truth. The use of the hamstring muscles and most of the gluteals in forcefully moving each leg backward during the ground contact phase is not the entire power story. Several other muscles can also be employed by adding power from the hips.

Most people walk with a rigid pelvis and fail to take advantage of the flexibility of this segment of the skeleton. To give you an idea of how flexible the pelvic skeleton can be, just visualize Elvis Presley in his heyday, or a belly dancer, or the popular dance of the sixties called the "twist." These examples illustrate how extremely flexible the pelvic girdle can be in different directions. By contrast, aerobic walking's flexibility is only moderate.

Aerobic walking technique moves one hip forward and the other back with each stride. The recovery leg and hip are brought forward, and the support leg and hip press backward. Both are strong movements. Most people find it easier to concentrate on the advancing hip to get the message from the brain to the working muscles, but some can focus better on the power of the ground-contact leg in overcoming the resistance of the ground. You can use you own best strategy to achieve the desired result—a 45-degree angle (as viewed from above) between the imaginary hip-to-hip line and the line of your body's forward direction (Figure 8).

Giraffe Legs? Or Chipmunk Quick?

The length of your stride may be too long, too short, or just right *for you.* Stride length is determined by how far your recovery leg comes forward to make ground contact, how far your support leg reaches back before toe off, and how much hip-line angulation

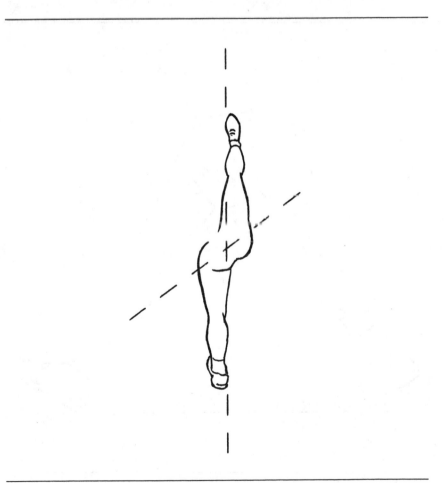

Figure 8. Top view of lower body.

(Figure 8) you use. The length of stride should be neither too restricted nor too stretched.

Visualize the angle that the legs form with the ground at heel contact and at toe off. If the angle at heel contact is too acute because you reached out with your leg for a very long stride, your muscles will be mechanically disadvantaged in trying to generate power to move your body forward (Figure 9). Conversely, if your stride is too short for the length of your legs, you will be losing inches on every stride (Figure 10).

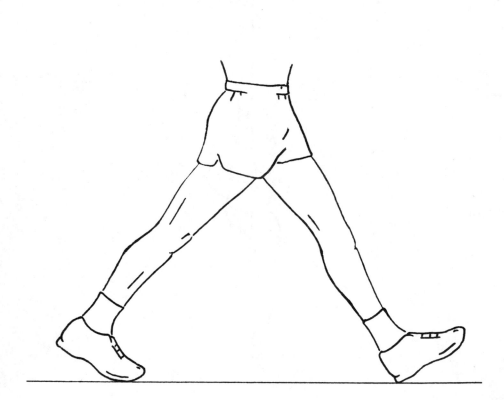

Figure 9. Stride length too long.

If you lengthen a too-short stride to optimum, yet keep the same stride rate, you will be going faster.

It is difficult to see yourself and to assess your own form. Better yet, ask a sharp-eyed walking friend for an unbiased opinion.

Force of Arms . . . or Balance?

In aerobic walking, the arms are bent 90 degrees at the elbows. If each arm is considered as a pendulum with its fixed point at the

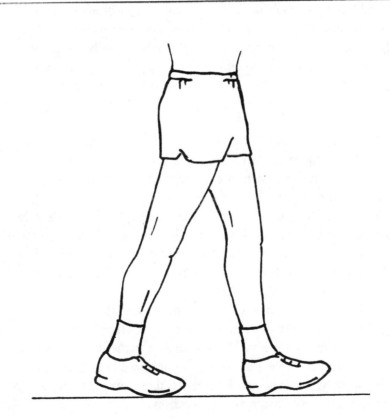

Figure 10. Stride length too short.

shoulder, a bent arm will be a shorter pendulum than a fully extended arm. A shorter pendulum, of course, swings faster than a long one (Figure 11).

When walking slowly, it is comfortable to have your arms swing at full length. But if you are walking at a good pace, arms bent at the elbow keep up with fast moving legs more easily. At high speed, you have little choice. As in running, you automatically bend the elbows because it feels right. If you tried to walk very fast with extended arms, you would soon reach a biomechanical limit to your pace.

With the arms bent at the elbow, there is a tendency to hunch the shoulders, and you may have to make a conscious effort to keep your shoulders relaxed. A hunched position, with its attendant muscle tightening, inhibits flexibility of the whole body. A good technique for relaxing the shoulders is to take a deep breath in and raise the shoulders; then let the shoulders completely fall as you exhale. Take note of how that relaxed position feels and keep it as you continue to walk.

With the arms bent at the elbow, the hands are held loosely, neither stretched open nor tightly fisted. The palm side of each hand faces inward; the back of each hand faces outward.

The path each hand describes as the arm swings is a slight arc toward the midline of the body. The hands should neither swing across the chest, nor punch out straight forward. Each arm swings as far back of the body as it swings forward, perhaps a little more so to balance the strong motion of the opposite leg that is trying to roll the earth around backward.

At first you may find it tiring to hold the arms at right angles. But you will gradually become stronger, and after a few weeks you will be able to maintain a 90-degree angle for the whole workout.

You have probably seen some exercise walkers pumping their arms vigorously. It is a widely held myth that pumping the arms will make the legs move faster and more powerfully and that you will burn up more calories with such arm motion. Next time you see such a walker, look carefully and you will note that the lower body is moving with no great vigor. The truth is that the legs drive the arms, not vice versa.

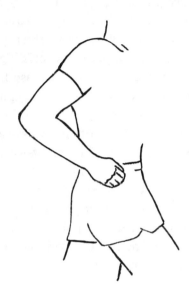

Figure 11. Arms bent at 90° angle.

As for burning calories, your arms are moved by relatively small muscles which are not working against the resistance of the earth, whereas your legs (in the Malkin Technique) use large muscles to move your entire body forward across the ground. It is the legs, not the arms, that can create significant metabolic change. Further, vigorous arm work will increase your respiratory rate and give you a false sense of workout intensity. As you progress toward aerobic levels in your walking program, you will use a scale of perceived exertion to judge workout intensity (See chapter 4). That estimate of perceived exertion will be more accurate if it reflects lower body work.

I advise allowing your arms to move in response to your legs and hips. (The key word here is *allowing*.) The longer and stronger your stride, the stronger your arm swing will be in response. The function of the arms, after all, is to provide a balance for the motion of the legs which are doing the real work of moving you forward.

It is not an easy balance: relaxed arms/shoulders and powerful legs/hips. You will need to concentrate on form for a few weeks until the muscles perform by habit. A helpful mind-body strategy is to dissociate the upper and lower halves of your body. First, walk in a relaxed fashion and take note of how the upper body feels. Then, keeping that easy arm and shoulder carriage, gradually increase the drive of your hips and legs. *Voila!* A fast and seemingly effortless pace.

So that no skeptical readers accuse me of overemphasizing technique, let me tell you about one of my walk training classes at the 92nd Street Y in New York City. The eight-week course is held each spring on a little used path in Central Park. Nearby, the main roadway is filled with runners, walkers, cyclists, and skaters. At the eighth session, our class went out among the proletariat on the roadway. One of the members of the group commented, "You know, the other walkers on the road seemed to be working so hard compared to us. But we went faster than most of them."

Posture

Aerobic walking form requires a tall, proud posture. Proper technique provides exercise to the lower back muscles and the abdominal muscles in a balanced fashion. This balance keeps the position of the spine and pelvis posture-perfect.

The good posture inherent in walking came into sharp focus for me a few years ago at the New York City Marathon. I was in the stands at the finish line taking notes for my column in the *Running News*. The column was to be on the walkers in the race, a race within a race, so to speak. I was able to spot each of the walkers among the masses of runners coming across the finish line. Bo Gustafson of Sweden was first in 3 hours, 19 minutes, followed over the next three hours by dozens of other walkers. The contrast between the runners and the walkers was striking. While some runners came in with a strong finish, many of them crossed under the digital clock in a state of imminent collapse. That year Rod Dixon of New Zealand came in first, crossing the finish line in 2:08:59 with his arms raised in victory. Geoff Smith of England, who had led for most of the race, was in pain the last half mile and fell to the ground as he crossed the finish line in second place. Many runners who followed had bowed bodies and bent heads even before the finish line.

The walkers were something else. Virtually all of them finished the 26.2 miles tall and proud looking. Posture had been hard-wired into their muscles and nerves by long practice.

With aerobic walking technique, you should feel that your head is held high, as if an angel is holding you up by the halo. Keep your shoulders relaxed. You will not become hump backed by relaxing your shoulders; your head held high will prevent that. The head is neither tilted up toward the sky nor down toward the ground. Rather, it should be balanced in line with your body's center of gravity. The feeling you will have when your form is proper is not that your head is a weight to be balanced atop your body, but that your head is helping to lift your body and keep your footsteps light.

In teaching aerobic walking, I watch carefully to see that my walkers neither lean back with the upper body nor lean forward by bending at the waist. Men tend to bend forward too much, and women who are models or dancers often lean back too far. If you bend forward from the waist, correct your posture by bringing your pelvis forward rather than bringing your shoulders back. If you tend to lean back too far with your upper body, think about your whole direction of movement being forward and upward.

Your chest and pelvis should equally lead you forward, and your center of gravity should be perfectly balanced over the supporting foot. The seeming dichotomy of a posture that is both straight and tall, yet relaxed, takes some time and concentration to achieve. But a few weeks is a short time for a lifetime exercise. Go for it!

Power Glide

Power and posture will get you to a good intermediate level of walking skill. To advance further you will need to add smoothness of technique to what you have already learned. It is a component of form that is difficult to analyze and difficult to learn by parts. Here, learning by wholes must be integrated with learning by parts.

The transition from one stride to the next must be very fluid, almost as if you are not taking separate footsteps. This gliding motion can be broken down into the following three components:

1. The transition between the toe-off of one stride and the heel contact of the next stride should be brief. That is, the amount of time that both feet are touching the ground should be as short as possible. The best way to achieve this transition is to abbreviate the end of the ground contact phase. Do not prolong the push off from the ball of the foot, and do not toe off at the very end. Merely end the ground contact phase early by starting to bring that foot forward for the new stride.

2. When you make ground contact with your heel at the very beginning of the support phase, make it a gentle contact.

3. Accelerate your speed gradually from the moment of heel strike and through the first two-thirds of each stride. Power production at heel strike is modest, greater when the leg is at vertical, and strongest when the leg is behind the body's center of gravity (Figure 12).

If your stride transition is fluid and the movement of your hips is flexible, your profile of motion will be one of gliding. The vertical level of your head will be constant, not up and down. It will be as if you were on a bicycle.

Whether you call the form floating, gliding, or rolling, it takes some concentration and some time to achieve. Be patient; be persistent. Learn by parts à la the three-step analysis above. Learn by wholes by imitating the overall form of a walker who exhibits this smooth style.

Smooth technique gives character to your walking form. It also raises the speed limit for your walking workouts. You will no longer be bound by the biomechanics of walking on two separate legs, a step at a time. Now you will feel as if your legs are part of a rotary engine instead of being piston rods.

Do you remember the story of my neighbors Rebecca and Marty? Rebecca was able to increase her speed by improving both stamina and technique. Marty, too, increased stamina, but without smooth technique he could not come close to matching his wife's

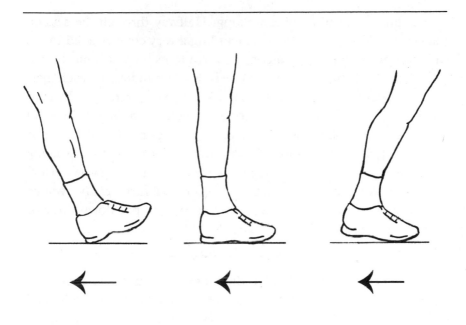

Figure 12. Gentle power at initial heel contact. Moderate power when leg is vertical. Greatest power when leg is behind body's center.

faster steps. Rebecca's fluid transfer of weight between strides allowed her to increase her stride turnover dramatically.

Rebecca's surge past her husband in walking ability is the rule rather than the exception. Women frequently surpass physically stronger men. I can offer examples from many walking clinics around the country. One, at the International Pedestrian Conference in Boulder, Colorado, is especially telling. In conjunction with my formal lecture, I led a participatory workshop in aerobic walking along a section of the celebrated Boulder Creek Trail. One of the participants was Dave, an avid hiker who leads walking tours in the Rockies. He is a rugged fellow who can walk the mountain trails for hours on end. Another in the workshop was Penny, a slim lady who walked for exercise but did not log even close to the weekly mileage that Dave turned out. But, Penny was a natural and quickly picked up the fluid form of aerobic walking. Halfway through the session she was breezing past everyone, including a very consternated Dave, who was pressing his separate-stride form to its biomechanical limit.

With smooth technique there is less pounding at each heel strike and less pressure on the hips, knees, and vertebrae. In running, the force exerted at every stride can be $2\frac{1}{2}$ to 5 times the weight of the body. At 150 pounds and running at a fair pace, each joint is subjected to a force of about 600 pounds at every footfall! Walking causes only $1\frac{1}{2}$ times body weight to be sustained at every stride. Smooth walking form reduces that pressure still further. That will be appreciated when you become strong enough to put down three or four miles of footsteps in a workout.

———————————

Technique is more than all the tangibles. It is also a challenge, and the mastery of the skill brings along with it a feeling of heightened self-esteem, even beyond the positive changes in brain chemistry.

CHAPTER 4

The Program
How Far, How Fast, How Often

Many people become surprisingly inquisitive when they come face to face with exercise. They ask not only how far, how fast, and how often, but also when, where, and if, and what about warmups and stretching, and hills and road surfaces, and many other details that are not relevant to the first week of workouts.

You do not need the genius of Joseph Heller to set yourself up for a Catch-22 scenario. If you are imaginative and looking for a reason not to work out, you can just say, "How can I exercise to get in shape if I'm not in shape to exercise?"

Then, there are the procrastination strategies:

o "I'll start exercising just as soon as I go on a diet. I need to lose ten pounds first."

o "I'll start walking outdoors as soon as the weather gets a little warmer."

o "As soon as the Easter holidays are over, I'm going to get rollerblades."

Ready to Start

The answer to creative avoidance is a simple question—"Can you walk for five minutes, turn around, and walk five minutes back?" That is all you need to start an effective walking program which will bring you health benefits and size/weight loss. You should be able to squeeze ten minutes from even a busy schedule and start today . . . or if there's a tornado today, tomorrow.

Some folks, whose efforts at rationalization elicit no sympathy, seek help from the medical profession. "But I have arthritis, you know." Or it may be sciatica, asthma, diabetes, heart disease, two left feet . . . . The truth is that none of these conditions should prevent you from starting a graduated walking program. In fact, walking improves most of them. Walking is a good part of taking care of many chronic conditions, even preventing them in the first place.

Medical Clearance

If you are young, have no symptoms of disease, and are free of cardiac risk factors, you won't need walking papers for a walk training program that starts with easy workouts. If you are not young and healthy, medical evaluation is advised. Consult your physician if:

o You are male and over forty, or female and over forty-five ✔

o At any age, you have chest pain with either exertion or emotional stress

o You have respiratory problems such as asthma

● You have high blood pressure

o You have cardiac risk factors such as high blood cholesterol or low HDL levels, a high-stress lifestyle, or a strong family history of heart disease

o You are pregnant, healthy or not

Tell your doctor that you wish to begin a graduated walking program, initially ten or fifteen minutes at a comfortable pace, three or four times a week. Your doctor will take a medical history and give you an examination, perhaps an EKG. When appropriate, an exercise stress test is done.

If you feel that by listening to your body you know everything about your needs and vulnerabilities, you are probably right in many instances. But there are also many cases of silent, significant pathology that can be identified only by medical testing. A checkup is advisable.

From all the caveats listed above, it may sound as if walk training is a risky business. If it is done by *gradually* working up to aerobic levels, you will incur little risk. The Eight-Week Program outlined at the end of this chapter, starting with short, easy workouts and gradually increasing distance and pace, will surely have your physician's blessing.

When to Walk

Is it better to walk in the morning or afternoon? Before or after dinner? During a full moon? How about the differences between Fridays and Mondays?

Nike™ has answered all these questions at once with its slogan, "Just Do It!" Consistency is more important than timing. But the question of when to exercise does have some influence on metabolism and motivation and is worth considering.

Are you a morning person or a night person? For early birds, morning workouts are best to take advantage of the time of day when adrenalin levels are rising. For night people, the thought of getting out of bed and moving purposefully enough to do a workout by 6:30 AM can cause them to faint back into a horizontal position.

Our work schedules and family commitments sometimes, or often, do not permit us to work out at times that are optimal for our personal metabolic cycles. Try to work out at whatever time is available. You will find that after a few weeks of "wrong time" workouts you won't be quite as confirmed an owl or lark as you thought you were. From a metabolic standpoint, human aerobic capacity is highest in the afternoon. You might conclude, then, that your performance would be better between 2 PM and 4 PM. It does not seem to work that way, however. One study found that the body's ability to use oxygen in the energy processes of muscle contraction was increased more than four percent between morning and afternoon (Munnings). Yet, maximum work levels were the same at both times of day. The body's ways are complex and enigmatic.

Body temperature parallels aerobic capacity and is highest in the afternoon. That diurnal variation plus the normal rise in body temperature during exercise can make hot summer afternoons a risky time to do outdoor exercise. In the summer, do your workouts in the morning or evening hours when the air is cooler.

In the winter, you need all the help you can get to keep warm. Sunny afternoons are best. There is even a school of exercise philosophy that considers temperatures below zero degrees Fahrenheit to be nature's way of advising, "Today, curl up with a good book to strengthen your emotional health. Tomorrow, you can look after your metabolism."

At lectures I am often asked whether it is better to exercise before or after meals. No one has ever asked whether to have lunch before or after exercise. Food is central, and exercise is scheduled around mealtime, if there is time. But regardless of whether food or exercise is your primary concern, the relationship between the two is a valid question.

Tips for Aerobic Walking in the AM. After a night's sleep, blood glucose levels are depressed—not a good condition to support a strong workout. Better to have an orange, a piece of toast, and a tall glass of water after arising. By the time you get washed, put on your workout suit, lace your shoes just right, and go outside, that small amount of food will be mostly digested. The carbohydrate from the orange and toast will be enough to bring your blood glucose to a daytime normal level but not enough to stimulate a large insulin release.

Tips for Aerobic Walking in the PM. For workouts at noon or later in the day, there is a question of whether to eat before your workout or sometime afterward. There have been studies showing that exercise shortly after a meal increases the energy cost of digestion—the thermic effect (Stamford). That sounds like an advantage if you are looking to burn more calories. However, a strong workout stops digestion as blood is diverted away from the gastrointestinal tract to the working muscles. The thermic effect would thus be cooled off. Besides, you never can do a good workout on a full stomach.

Having lunch or dinner after exercise has the further advantage that your appetite is held down while you are enjoying the afterglow of the workout. This phenomenon of post-exercise appetite suppression is observed consistently by nearly every endurance athlete.

Air Quality. Another factor to count in the timing of exercise is air pollution. Air pollution comes in the forms of ground level ozone and auto emissions.

Ozone is generally lowest in the early morning and late afternoon when sunlight is weakest. The weather bureau announces ozone alerts on days of danger. If your respiratory or cardiovascular system is compromised, please heed such alerts.

Auto exhaust gases contain carbon monoxide, which is especially dangerous if you are working out and breathing more deeply than at rest. A study done in Manhattan along the East River Drive during rush hour showed higher levels of carbon monoxide-bound hemoglobin in runners than in people who were were standing or strolling (Nicholson). In the city it is better to work out well before or after rush hour and at locations where mean-spirited drivers will not get you with their bumpers or their tailpipes.

Where to Walk

Trees are far better environmental companions than cars. They are esthetically pleasant and they gift you with oxygen. Parks should be your first choice for aerobic walking.

Surfaces. In my own workouts I used to pay little attention to surfaces, relying on fluid technique to soften the effect of even a hard road surface. Then I experienced the concrete of the Boulder Creek Trail in Boulder, Colorado. It is a pedestrian-and-bicycle path that runs alongside Boulder Creek right through the entire city. As a speaker at the International Pedestrian Conference who espoused the use of legs as a prime means of transportation, I used the trail to walk to and from the Conference Center each day for three days. I was practicing what I preached.

On the first day I wore sneakers with a fair amount of cushioning. The next day I wore sneakers that were very thin-soled to demonstrate that cushioning could come from walking technique. The third day, I felt the accumulated impacts in the form of tender metatarsals. It was a learning experience twice over. I learned that surface can make a difference even for experienced walkers, and I learned that I didn't know it all in the first place.

Now more aware of surface quality, I find the best to be the artificial material used for high school and college outdoor tracks. A second best is an unpaved country road if it is level and free of rocks and potholes. An asphalt surface is harder, yet not all that bad on the feet. Concrete, as noted above, calls for well-cushioned sneakers as well as fluid form.

Uphills and Downhills. My friend Dick lives in the upper Delaware River valley. He is an avid walker who has long felt that walking on a level trail did not give him an adequate workout. He always welcomed a long uphill in any of his workouts so that he would have to work harder. He is fortunate that the area in which he lives has many trails that seem to go only uphill. One year, Dick and I scheduled a monthly series of River Walks, inviting anyone in the area to join us. On these walks I gave Dick occasional instruction in technique, and after a while he was able to achieve a faster stride. Toward the end of the series, he was able to get a good workout without, as he described it, "charging the hills."

For beginning walkers it is best to start out on fairly level terrain. There are enough matters of form to think about without dealing with ups and downs.

For advanced walkers who walk on varied terrain, there are a few simple rules of posture for walking upgrades, downgrades, and on the flat.

o On level terrain, your body should be perpendicular to the ground, in line with gravity (Figure 13).

o On uphills, there is a tendency to bend forward at the waist, which stresses the lower back muscles, shortens the stride, and prevents a smooth transition between strides. Instead, keep the same tall, relaxed posture and stay in line with gravity, rather than with the surface of the trail. You will lean forward a little, but do not bend at the waist (Figure 14).

o On downgrades, do not lean back; rather, keep your body tall and perpendicular to the surface. Being perpendicular to a downhill trail, you will lean forward with respect to gravity (Figure 15).

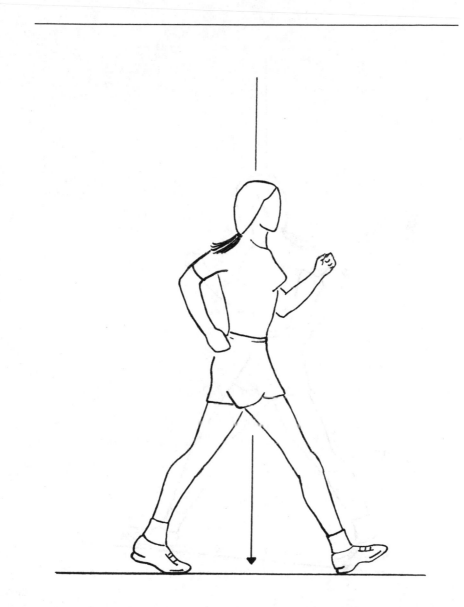

Figure 13.

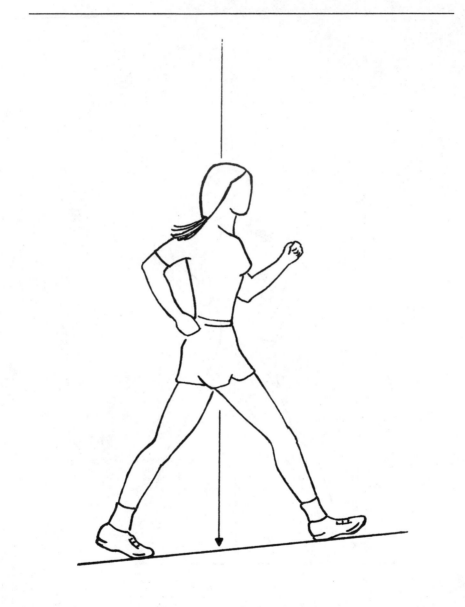

Figure 14.

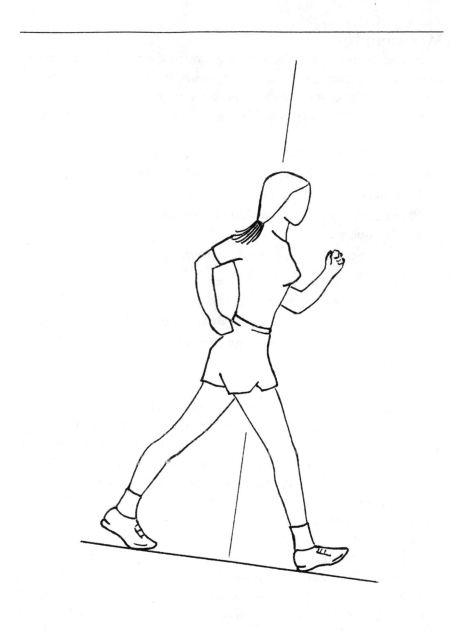

Figure 15.

Warming Up

The purpose of a warmup is to warm the muscles that will be used in the workout to follow. Pretty simple. Yet, if we take the exercise of walking, it turns out that dozens of different muscles are used. To warm up every one, it would take many different calisthenic routines.

Let's step back from focusing on specific muscles and look at the body's overall temperature physiology. We know that:

1. External heat increases body temperature.
2. Physical massage increases blood flow and temperature of the tissues touched.
3. Rhythmic contraction of muscles increases blood flow and temperature of those muscles.

Now we have some answers:

1. You can warm up the whole body in a hot tub.
2. You can bring along a massage therapist to work on your walking muscles.
3. You can walk at less than workout pace for a few minutes.

The first two types of warmup seem to be wonderful choices, but each is likely to become a pleasantly extended warmup, followed by no workout at all. The third—using the same exercise you will use in the workout, but at a slower pace—is the best choice. It is also the most effective way to increase blood flow to the muscles that will be doing the work. You will not have to worry about missing a small muscle group as you would if you were using a supposedly comprehensive calisthenic routine.

Increasing the physical temperature of the muscle fibers decreases their viscosity, making them more pliable. Theoretically, this elimination of stiffness should lessen the risk of injury, but so far a protective effect from warming up has not been confirmed by data. My prudent grandmother offers her wisdom: "Maybe it wouldn't help, but it wouldn't hurt either."

Other reasons for warming up have a more medically acceptable basis:

○ Increasing the blood supply to the muscles provides them with more oxygen and glucose and so enables you to establish a strong, steady pace early in the workout.

○ The hemoglobin of warmer blood releases its oxygen to the muscle tissues more easily. A similarly enhanced release of oxygen occurs in warm myoglobin, the oxygen carrying molecule found in muscle fibers.

○ The pacemaker tissues of the heart are protected from the rhythm disturbances that have been observed in exercise from a cold start.

The findings of R. James Barnard and his research team at UCLA School of Medicine are noteworthy. Their subjects were ten healthy males, ages 20 to 52, with no evidence of heart disease. The men ran on a treadmill at maximal effort (10 mph at a 24 percent grade) in two trials—one with a warmup and one without a warmup. The sudden exertion without a warmup produced abnormal electrocardiographic changes in six of the ten subjects, three of them severe enough to indicate significant constriction of the blood supply (ischemia) to the heart muscle. With a warmup, only two of the ten exhibited EKG changes upon maximal exercise, and these changes were minor.

○ Warming up, which increases blood flow to the brain, improves mood and reduces any reluctance towards working out.

How Often?

Frequency is an easy prescription: Work out one day and rest the next day. Then repeat the cycle and continue forever. You can start your three or four workouts per week immediately. You do not have to build up to this frequency. The three or four workouts should be spaced fairly evenly across the week. If your life is busy, "fairly evenly" allows you to work out two days back to back, or to make up for two inactive days by doing a somewhat longer workout on the next day. It does not condone five days of sloth during the week followed by two workouts on Saturday and another two on

Sunday. That is a prescription for metabolic mischief and musculoskeletal distress.

There is good reason for resting 48 hours between workouts. Muscle glycogen is used for energy needs in your workout and becomes depleted. The replenishing process takes about two days. Studies of runners and swimmers have confirmed that strong workouts on consecutive days cause progressive depletion of muscle glycogen. The process of restoring glycogen levels can not be rushed, not by pasta primavera, not even by a generous helping of pecan pie.

Muscle protein is another concern. It is well known that the proteins of the body are in a dynamic state of equilibrium. Ongoing synthesis and degradation occur as a function of life, regardless of whether you live well or badly. During exercise, protein building is depressed. Forty-eight hours of rest after exercise assures that protein balance is restored. In addition, it takes 48 hours between strong workouts for lactic acid and other metabolic byproducts of exercise to be cleared from the working muscles.

For those who need the discipline of a scheduled workout every day, I advise a strong workout on day one, an easy form-polishing workout on day two, another strong workout on day three, and so on.

How Far?

Measuring your workout in terms of distance presents some problems. Most walking paths are not measured in miles. Those that are exactly measured, such as school tracks, are only one-quarter mile (or 400 meters) in length which requires a great deal of going around in circles for a 45-minute workout. For most folks, it is easy to lose track of the number of laps completed. I know that when I am concentrating on form and pace, I can count about four laps. Then I am not sure if it is the fifth lap coming up or if I have already done five.

The best way to measure distance is with a wristwatch. Measuring distance in terms of time is convenient, easy, and metabolically accurate. The aerobic threshold for exercise is between 30 and 60 minutes, depending on the choice of exercise and the intensity. For walking at a brisk pace, the aerobic threshold time is about 45 minutes.

Caution: Unless you are already highly fit, do not start your walking program at threshold levels. Fifteen minutes is sufficient for each of the first week's workouts. Then, gradually work up to 45 minutes. If you are already fit, you may need only three or four weeks to reach aerobic levels of distance and speed. If you are unfit you may need eight to twelve weeks to get to aerobic levels. Medically compromised individuals may need a few weeks longer.

Although walking is easy and safe, it can be a serious exercise and, as such, is worthy of respect.

Stephanie is an owner of the health spa where I teach aerobic walking on occasional weekends. On my first weekend there, I instructed the guests and the staff, Stephanie included. Steph leads many of the hikes, often ten miles and more, snowshoes over difficult terrain in the winter, and challenges her rock-climbing skills on the cliffs of the nearby Shawangunk Mountains. She is physically tough and mentally determined. On the first day of instruction in aerobic walking technique, she picked up the basic form and was able to move along at a fast pace. Thirty-five minutes later she was almost exhausted and said breathlessly, "That's it. That's a full workout." And it was! She was using different muscles for aerobic walking than she used in hiking and running. Over the weeks that followed, further practice in aerobic walking increased her endurance substantially, and now she can easily do five miles at a strong pace.

Violet, a student in another walking program, is a senior citizen who was barely capable of walking ten minutes when she started. Yet, Violet increased her workout time to 45 minutes over a period of twelve weeks. The human body is capable of notable feats if the training is consistent and the increases in distance and pace are gradual.

There are individual differences among people in how much they drive themselves in their exercise training. Stephanie quickly shifts into overdrive, but Violet tends to fall into a comfortable pace and rhythm. At one point I felt Violet ought to increase her workout distance to compensate for the lower intensity.

I suggested, "Violet, you're getting to be a much stronger walker now, and I think you can increase one of your workouts each week to a full hour instead of 45 minutes."

She replied, "Oh, but it takes me a whole hour to do a 45-minute workout."

Violet's hour was a metaphor to let me know that she was working hard at her chosen exercise.

Each of us is unique, not only in personality but in physiology as well. Each will have somewhat different workout time requirements to achieve maximum benefit. Still, there are minimums and maximums to be kept in mind.

If you wish to increase your workout time beyond 45 minutes, it is all right up to a point. That point seems to be about 90 minutes. Beyond 90 minutes at a strong pace is tempting the gremlins of the overtraining syndrome. These dangers—musculoskeletal injury and physiological dysfunction—are discussed more fully in chapter 9, "Safely, Safely."

Decreasing workout time tempts the fates in the opposite way. If your workout is less than 40 minutes, it approaches the aerobic threshold for distance. Below that threshold, your body will not respond metabolically to your efforts. Better to leave a small margin of safety and work out for 45 minutes.

How Fast?

Just as you were advised to begin your walking program at less than aerobic distance, so you should begin at a nice easy pace. Over the course of a few weeks you will gradually increase speed until you reach your personal aerobic threshold. Most people achieve this pace within eight weeks. Just be patient and do not rush into speedy workouts too soon.

Miles Per Hour

There are different ways to measure speed. Miles per hour (or minutes per mile) is a common enough measure for foot travel, but a measured mile is required to be accurate. Measuring speed in miles per hour also tends to create standards that are appropriate for only the statistically average individual. How many of us are average?

An athletic whippet of a man who works out three or four times a week can move twice as fast as a couch potato whose most challenging exercise is emptying a bowl of buttered popcorn while watching a movie. Not only is the whippet *able* to go faster, he *needs* to go faster to reach the aerobic threshold that creates or maintains metabolic change for his body. Aerobic threshold depends on:

1. Current state of fitness
2. Size
3. Cardiovascular health
4. Efficiency of walking technique

It is better to set your pace by the needs of your own body rather than by the needs of an average body.

I can give you a few guidelines in terms of minutes per mile, but remember, they are only guidelines. In the average middle aged, sedentary female who is basically healthy, 14 to 15 minutes per mile for 45 minutes are usually the thresholds for metabolic change. For the young, athletic, and healthy individual—male or female—12 to 13 minutes per mile is the threshold. Older, medically compromised, or frail individuals will benefit at even slower speeds.

The bottom line is the amount of effort that you as an individual put into your workout.

Target Heart Rate

Physical effort—musculoskeletal work—drives the heart to pump faster and stronger. As the level of exercise intensity is raised, the heart rate increases in an attempt to pump more blood to the working muscles. With a continued increase in exercise intensity, the heart rate reaches its limit.

Heart rate is easy to measure—high tech with a pulse monitor, or low tech with your fingers. You can determine the exact number of beats per minute and compare that number to a standard. Very neat.

For an exercise to be "aerobic" the intensity must be above a workout speed that drives your heart rate to 60 percent of maximal. Aerobic intensity must also be below a heart rate of 85 percent of maximal. At less than the 60 to 85 percent range, the exercise is too mild and a training effect does not occur. Above that range, the effort becomes anaerobic and your muscles go into oxygen debt. So far, so good.

But if everyone's target heart rate is to be measured scientifically as a percentage of maximal heart rate, everyone has to be tested for maximum. The scientists, in an attempt to finesse this problem, tested a sampling of people and devised a formula they thought was suitable for the average body: 220 minus age, multiplied by 60 percent to 85 percent equals target heart rate range.

If it seemed too easy, it was. Some exercise physiologists found that the formula-predicted maximal heart rates and the actually-measured maximal heart rates were often quite different. Other investigators found a wide dispersion of treadmill-measured maximums for every age group they examined. Cardiologists found that many cardiac patients could not come close to reaching a formula-based maximum.

A further source of inaccuracy is inherent in the testing procedure for maximal heart rate. In the treadmill test, maximal heart rate is recorded as the heart rate at the point of volitional exhaustion. One person may consider himself or herself exhausted after little exercise; another who is more stoic may push on with greater effort before pronouncing exhaustion.

Also, different muscle groups provide different amounts of stimulus to the heart. Small-muscle exercise, such as arm work, produces a higher heart rate than large-muscle exercise, such as leg work.

The difference between weight-bearing and non-weight-bearing exercise introduces another confounding factor.

All told, target heart rate has clear and present limitations as a guide to intensity of exercise.

Perception of Effort

In the early sixties, Gunnar Borg of the University of Stockholm proposed and proved that the individual's own perception of effort can be used to monitor the pace of an aerobic workout. Borg's scale reads from 6 to 20 (Figure 16).

Effort	Numeric Value
Very, very light	6 to 7
Light	8 to 11
Moderate	12
Moderate to hard—*aerobic zone*	13 to 14
Hard	15
Very hard	16 to 18
All out effort	19 to 20

Figure 16. Borg Scale of Perceived Exertion.

When exercising at 13 to 14, "moderate to hard," working muscles are using oxygen at proper aerobic levels—the so-called aerobic zone. The correlation between the subjective measure of perceived exertion and the objective standards of oxygen utilization is remarkably consistent.

In aerobic walking clinics, I use perception of effort in setting pace for individual participants. I have also found other descriptive guides to add to "somewhat hard" in targeting the 13-to-14 level on Borg's scale.

o You should be a little out of breath (not a lot) throughout your workout.

o You should feel that you are pressing your pace a little, that you are making an effort.

o You should find it difficult to hold an easy conversation with a walking partner. You should be able to speak only in short phrases, not long sentences.

o You should feel you can maintain your pace only as long as your planned workout. You should have no substantial reserve left at the end; nor should you give out before the end.

In the research community the question arose, "How could such soft science be so precise?" Various investigators tried to find the answer by looking at the biological factors that contribute to an athlete's sense of effort. They examined relative oxygen demand, respiratory rate and effort, muscle fatigue, blood pH, lactic acid levels, heart rate, cardiac output, and psychological factors. Interaction between and among factors was the rule, but lactic acid levels seemed to be the most significant indicator of effort.

Out of the complexity came a clear basic concept: The human brain is capable of integrating data from many tissues, organs, and systems and can read the body's degree of effort with exquisite accuracy.

It is not 100 percent foolproof. Small differences exist between trained and untrained individuals. There are also some minor differences between men and women and differences between exercising on a treadmill and exercising on an outdoor track. But perceived exertion remains the most accurate, easiest to use, and most personalized measure of exercise intensity. Use it in, and for, good health.

Interval Training

A steady pace above aerobic threshold and below anaerobic threshold assures the health changes described in the previous chapters.

For rhythm and constancy, a steady pace is fine. For challenge and variety, you can combine fast and slow segments in a workout and achieve the same overall metabolic change. This method is called *interval training.*

Interval training consists of dividing a workout into cycles of fast and slow sections, each of the proper length. For example, a cycle of a fast five minutes followed by a slow three minutes, repeated five times, would be equal to a 40-minute workout at a constant speed. The fast segments are not at all-out speed, but they are at a faster pace than possible for the entire workout.

You can vary the intervals from a minimum of a quarter mile to a maximum of one mile. Studies with runners have shown that intervals of less than two minutes for the fast segments are not efficient in improving aerobic capacity.

Interval training is a good way to increase level of fitness and to break out of a plateau. It is not, however, for novices. After attaining a good level of fitness, select any interval from two to ten minutes at a fast pace followed by a slow interval for about half that amount of time. Repeat the cycle until the total time is 40 to 50 minutes.

You may mix interval training with exercising at a constant pace, but no fair doing five minutes at your regular speed followed by a slow three minutes. A workout is a workout.

Thresholds of Frequency, Distance, and Speed

The recommendations for how often, how far, and how fast and are determined by the body's threshold needs. If you exercise only once or twice a week *or* less than 40 to 50 minutes per workout *or* at a leisurely to moderate pace, your metabolism will not change. You must achieve all three thresholds to trigger the biological changes noted in chapter 2. These are not my rules. I am only reporting your body's own rules.

Cooling Down

The human body does not like abrupt change. This physiologic rule is enough reason to ease out of a workout instead of stopping abruptly. There is another, more specific reason for walking around for a few minutes after a workout. During the workout, the heart is beating fast and strong; cardiac output is high. The muscles of the body, especially the legs, are contracting rhythmically to move you along at a nice pace. At the same time, they are acting as a supplemental pump to help move the blood in the veins of the lower body back to the heart.

At the end of a workout, the heart slows down gradually, not suddenly. If you were to stand still at the end of a workout, the venous blood returning to the heart from the lower body would slow down abruptly. The heart then might receive too little blood to provide an adequate supply to the brain and other vital organs.

Cooling down with easy walking also serves to eliminate lactic acid and other metabolites, not only from the blood but from the muscles that generated these by-products during workout. All that is required is a continued rhythmic contraction of the muscles to bring a fresh supply of oxygenated blood to those muscles.

Cooling down for aerobic walking workouts is done in exactly the same way as warming up. Walk at a slower pace for a few minutes until the heart rate approaches a normal (nonexercise) rate.

Stretching

After the muscles have contracted rhythmically a few thousand times during a workout, they become sensitized. If a sensitized muscle is allowed to shorten, it may contract as powerfully as it did during the workout. Shortening of muscles can occur just by sitting in a cramped position or moving a limb in an unaccustomed way. Such a contraction feels like a severe spasm, not just a minor cramp. The purpose of stretching is to lengthen the hair-trigger muscles gently and hold them at length until they relax. Thirty seconds per stretch is usually sufficient.

Walking may seem to be an exercise which hardly deserves precautions such as stretching, but aerobic walking technique is not just brisk walking. The hamstring muscles are used powerfully and do need to be stretched. The calf muscles and the back muscles also work hard and can use the stretching. Stretching is a physiological need.

Three specific stretches are advised after an aerobic walking workout. The general rules that apply to these stretches are simple and sensible. Go into each stretch gradually, hold the stretch passively for thirty seconds (without bouncing), and then come out of the stretch gradually.

Stretch 1

Calf muscles get a fair amount of work even when you follow proper form and do not push off from the ball of the foot and big toe at the end of the stride. This is the stretch that runners often do, pressing their hands against a wall or tree, one foot forward and one foot back. Here are the basics:

o The forward foot is placed one-half a foot length from the wall (or lamppost, tree, or partner). The other foot is placed about three foot lengths back with the entire foot (heel, too) touching the ground. The back foot should point straight ahead. The calf muscles of the back leg will be stretched; the front leg is used only for support. Hands touch the wall gently with elbows slightly bent. The forward knee bends, and hips move forward with the back heel remaining in contact with the ground. The upper body is erect, not bent forward in an attempt to press the shoulders toward the wall.

o The stretching should be felt in the calf muscles of the back leg, but should not be extreme to the point of pain. If the calf muscles are being stretched excessively, move the back foot a little further forward.

o Hold the position for 30 seconds. Release the stretch gradually by slowly moving away from the wall.

Note these fine points:

o The position of the lower part of the front leg (from the knee down) should be vertical.

o The knee of the back leg can be slightly bent, still keeping the heel in contact with the ground. The more the knee is bent, the more the lower muscle group of the calf will be stretched. The straighter the knee, the more the upper muscle group of the calf will be stretched.

o Do not try to push the wall, tree, or your partner down; use for balance only (Figure 17).

Stretch 2

The use of the arms in aerobic walking technique may be less than vigorous, but a few thousand swings during a workout does give the upper back muscles a significant amount of exercise. They deserve some attention.

o   With each arm bent, place the palm of each hand on the opposite elbow. Let the shoulders relax and bend the head and shoulders forward with chin close to chest.

o   Hold the stretch for 30 seconds, and release slowly.

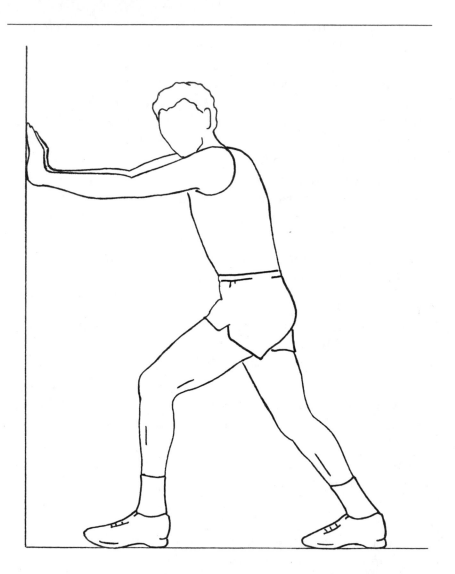

Figure 17.

Note these fine points:

o   The forward bend is from the neck and shoulders, not at the waist.

o   Do not hunch the shoulders; rather, allow them to fall into a
    relaxed position (Figure 18).

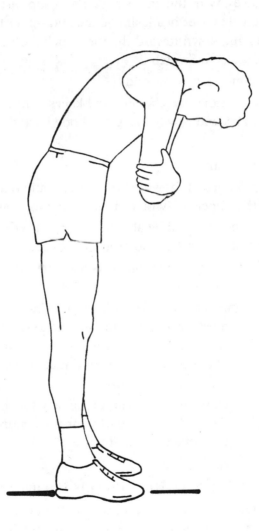

Figure 18.

Stretch 3

The hamstring, gluteal, and lower back muscles supply power for forward propulsion in aerobic walking. They are called upon to perform at a high percentage of their maximum power output, and they deserve some TLC. Stretching is in order.

o   Bend slightly at the knees and waist and place hands on thighs near the knees. With the hands acting as a support for the upper body, gradually lower head, shoulders, and upper body; then let the hands hang down toward the toes. Tuck the head in, chin close to chest as in Stretch 2.

o   Hold the stretch for 30 seconds.

o   To come out of the stretch, bend the knees a little, place hands back on thighs, and slowly bring the body back to a standing position.

Note these fine points:

o   Do not forcibly reach down to your toes. Rather, allow only the weight of the upper body to keep you hanging down.

o   As you breathe, you will be able to lower your arms and shoulders a little closer to the ground with each exhalation.

o   Balance your weight evenly on heels and toes—not too far forward and not too far back.

o   Bending the knees a little more allows your hands to reach lower and provides more stretching for the lower back muscles. Straightening the knees stretches the hamstrings more. You will be able to find the degree of knee bend that allows equal stretching for both muscle groups.

o   If you are so flexible that you can practically touch the palms of your hands to the ground, just curl your fingers up a bit so your wrists are closest to the ground (Figure 19).

Stretching: How Much Is Enough?

Right after a workout and cool down, you need only one set of stretches. If the workout was strong, it is advisable to repeat the

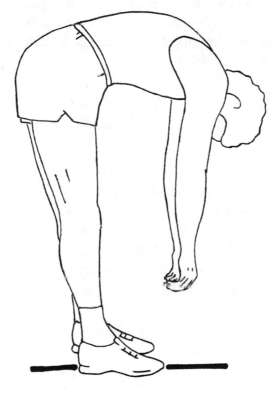

Figure 19.

stretches later in the day and the next day. Be sure to walk around for a couple of minutes to warm the muscles before the repeat stretches. Stretching cold muscles can cause microtears in muscle fibers.

A few walkers have told me that their muscles need more than 30 seconds per stretch. No problem. Even a couple of minutes is fine if the stretch is gentle.

You may also wish to stretch other muscle groups after the required three stretches. Stretch as much as you feel you need. In fact, two other muscle groups that get a little work in aerobic walking—the psoas muscle of the groin and the quadriceps muscles of the front of the thigh—can benefit from stretching.

For all stretches, the muscles should be held at length without rebounding for at least 30 seconds.

Eight-Week Aerobic Walking Program

Before each workout, warm up. Use the Malkin Technique throughout the workout. Afterward, cool down and stretch. The following schedule is somewhat flexible. If you are fit and healthy, you may start with Week Two. If you have significant medical problems, you should consult with your doctor and may start with five- or ten-minute workouts every other day to prepare for Week One.

Week One: 15 minutes at a gentle pace, every other day

Week Two: 20 minutes at a comfortable pace (slightly faster than "gentle"), every other day

Week Three: 25 minutes at a moderate pace (slightly faster than "comfortable"), every other day

Week Four: 30 minutes at a somewhat brisk pace (slightly faster than "moderate"), every other day

Week Five: 35 minutes at a brisk pace, every other day

Week Six: 40 minutes at a brisk pace, every other day

Week Seven: 45 minutes at a brisk pace, every other day

Weeks Eight through 5,000: 45 minutes at a very brisk pace, every other day

You will notice changes in your size and shape, a rise in your energy levels, and other indications of metabolic change—all occurring sometime between Week Six and Week Eight. These signs of metabolic magic will encourage you to make aerobic walking a part of your lifestyle. As you go on forever, the esthetic and health benefits will reach new heights, and you will be delighted by your continued progress.

CHAPTER 5

Heads, You Win
The Art and Science of Exercise Motivation

Erma Bombeck claims to have lost 250 pounds in two years. The first two weeks she lost 10 pounds. The second two weeks she gained 11 pounds back. The third week she lost; the fourth week she gained. And so it went for two years. At the end of that time she had lost 250 pounds and gained 260 pounds.

Erma Bombeck is not unique in being able to lose so much weight nor in being able to gain it all back again. She is just funnier than other dieters in telling about it. Most dieters—90 percent and more—are not successful at becoming and staying slim. The reasons have less to do with diet than with lack of proficient exercise. The exercise, of course, is not effective if it is done sporadically or every so seldom. Enter motivation. Motivation is needed to exercise regularly just as for many other activities in life.

The Motivation Model

A number of investigators have looked into the art and science of motivation and have tried to apply what they have learned to encourage exercise. Roy J. Shephard of the University of Toronto has created a model for motivation that correlates beliefs, behavior, and attitude.

Belief

Belief underlies everything. We are not likely to do something we perceive as unpleasant and/or ineffective. But just because we believe in a particular concept or activity does not necessarily mean we will be moved to action. For example, most people believe that exercise is good for their health, but far fewer are motivated enough to exercise regularly.

Rod K. Dishman of the University of Georgia has reviewed different models of exercise motivation. Two of the models seem useful for aerobic walking.

1. The model of self-efficacy is simple. You have to believe you are capable of performing the activity before you will do it. If you never learned to swim, you will not be highly motivated to swim at aerobic distance and pace. Walking, on the other hand, fits this theory well—everyone has the skills to start a walking program.

2. The self-esteem model of exercise notes that exercise heightens self-esteem and higher self-esteem reinforces exercise. With this positive cycle, you will begin to believe that you will succeed in losing size and weight permanently.

These models are not pure belief theory. Behavior and attitude always interact with belief, and our actions (or inaction) are not always predictable. Yet, it is worthwhile using any psychological tools that help to make exercise a regular part of our lifestyles. Take an active part in developing a positive belief system. Belief strategies as simple as selecting an exercise that is not intimidating will raise motivation levels.

Behavior

Behavior changes can increase the incentive to exercise by making it easy to start—and easy to continue. Behavioral strategies can bring about positive change in our activities through the use of psychosocial learning principles, such as visual reminders, setting aside priority time for an activity, and involving an amiable person in the activity with you.

Attitude

Attitude is the real force behind what we do or don't do. I define attitude broadly. Attitude includes:

o Sense of self
o Personality
o Self-image
o Societal norms or, more simply, peer influence
o Energy levels
o Self-expectation
o Emotional state

While behavioral strategies address the influence of external factors on motivation and behavior, attitude, taken broadly, deals with internal controls. Attitude is not immutable. Events, experience, and insight can change attitude. You can use a few attitude-betterment tactics such as using a physical warmup for mood elevation when you don't feel like doing a workout, or wearing an outfit that gives you the look of an athlete.

Personality studies have shown that Type A individuals (driving, impatient, anger-reactive) respond well to psychological training for increasing exercise levels. Type B individuals (more stable, less intense, less reactive) are not as responsive to such strategies. Internal motivation can work well for Type B people who feel the need to exercise for either esthetic or health reasons. If, however, a Type B person is convinced that he or she is not athletic, that attitude can block motivation.

My neighbor Maurice, a physician, recently had a heart attack. After a few weeks when he was well on the way to recovery and back to work on a part-time basis, I offered him a walking lesson. As an internist-cardiologist, Maurice knows that aerobic exercise will reduce his risk of another heart attack. Yet he politely declined the offer, saying, "Well, you know, Mort, I'm more the cerebral type than the athletic type." Maurice's self-image is blocking his medical logic.

Beyond personality, the elements of mood and emotion strongly influence motivation. Research has shown, for example, that obese individuals have less control over negative emotions. That is a chicken and egg situation, of course. Did the diminished control lead to obesity, or does obesity lead to a sense of hopelessness? Probably both. It has also been observed that success in weight loss is inversely related to severity of depression. Mood and emotion can make a difference in exercise motivation as well as in weight loss.

We can use the three factors—belief, behavior, and attitude—in positive ways to exercise regularly.

The Ways and Means of Motivation

Enough theory! Now it is time for practical ways of starting to walk for exercise and continuing for a long, healthy lifetime. Pick the motivation strategies from the list below that can work for you, and just do them.

Can Do

You have known from the age of two how to place one foot after the other. You already know the basics of walking. If you can step outside the front door, walk five minutes down the street, and return, you can start an aerobic walking program.

I have come across many individuals who considered themselves total athletic incompetents, yet were able to become skilled walkers. Joe is a good example. For his entire life—25 years in England and the last 15 in the United States—he never did anything more athletic than lift a pint of ale in a pub. Within the first four weeks of an eight-week walking course, Joe discovered he had a talent for aerobic walking. By the last two sessions he had become so good that he was leaving the rest of the group in his jet stream right from the start and lapping everyone at least once by the end of the 45-minute workout on a 600-yard track. He and I were both elated.

Whether you are athletic or not, you can become a strong walker. That achievement will be powerful motivation for you to make aerobic walking part of your lifestyle.

Finding a Friendly Exercise

Select an exercise that is not scary. Walking is less intimidating than lacrosse or boxing. It is neither dangerous nor aggressive; in fact, it creates a feeling of peace and a sense of democracy. Having to move under your own leg power without a three-pointed star or leaping jaguar to lead the way is a powerful equalizer. It is hard to be angry toward another walker who is sharing the same earth and contributing to a syncopation of stride rhythms. Such feelings of amity will encourage you to count walking as your primary exercise.

Safekeeping

Avoiding injury will prevent pain, disability, and medical bills. It is also an important motivational factor. If you become injured from an exercise, you may wonder, "If exercise is supposed to make me healthy, what am I doing in a doctor's office?" After you recover, the inertia of a few sedentary weeks may lead you to rationalize that your body is too fragile for exercise. By selecting walking—the safest exercise—you will avoid the risk of injury *and* the excuse for not exercising.

Walking as Good Medicine

Walking is beneficial for a number of medical conditions from hypertension to osteoporosis to diabetes. (See chapter 7 for a more extensive listing.) Physicians are in agreement and endorse walking as exercise. If you have any medical condition, discuss your walking program with your doctor and obtain his or her accord. When you start looking good and feeling good, your physician may think, "That was a great idea I had—to prescribe walking."

You can smile and say, "Thanks, Doc." And your motivation will be reinforced.

Walking in Good Company

For most people, having company is good motivation. When going out for a solo workout, it is easy to say to yourself, "It's kind of windy; maybe I'll wait until tomorrow." But if you are meeting a walking partner or group, you will be more inclined to work out at the appointed time. Sometimes we need company, and other times we need solitude—enjoy a mix of workouts.

When you have a partner for a workout, you each may have a different pace. But you can go to the park and warm up together. Then, you can work out individually and, afterward, cool down, stretch, and go home together.

There are other variations. My friend, Belinda, occasionally joins me for a workout on the $\frac{7}{8}$-mile oval in Marine Park in Brooklyn. We walk in opposite directions and have a chance to smile or offer a thumbs up sign twice every loop.

Company can also come unsolicited. In Alley Pond Park in Queens, New York, there is an old right-of-way called the Vanderbilt Parkway that runs eastward for a few miles. Motor vehicles are banned, leaving the delightful, tree-shaded trail to cyclists and pedestrians. It is also a haven for many species of birds. The crows who flock there always let you know of their presence, "Kaw! Kaw! Kaw!" Violet, a former teacher who walks there regularly, thinks of them as dyslexic coaches calling, "Walk! Walk! Walk!"

Stepping Out in Fashion

Walking provides the greatest latitude in choice of clothing and equipment. You can find high-tech walking and running shoes with every conceivable system for cushioning, lateral support, flexion, and lacing. Technology has also produced special fibers and weaves for socks, undergarments, overgarments, and accessories to keep you cool, warm, ventilated, and visible. And, they come in every color ever and never imagined on the day the Creator said, "Let there be light."

Of course you can do as well with a pair of plain but comfortable sneakers and an old, gray sweatsuit. Low-tech, antifashion can be a personal statement in itself. In walking, it is form, not fashion, that equals function. If you are an exceptional walker, your style will overshadow all the accoutrements.

Although we know that beauty is inherent in the elegant functioning of the musculoskeletal system, many of us also have favorite workout clothes. If you have a favorite color or a special outfit that makes you feel more like an athlete, or a T-shirt from a particular event, it can add to your overall motivation. Motivation can always use a little extra help.

Walking as an Ally Against Fat

People, from ancient times until today, have been guided by the adage, "The enemy of my enemy is my friend."

You can use that concept to increase exercise motivation. First, consider excessive fat as your enemy. Fat already knows that exercise is its enemy. It follows that exercise, the enemy of your enemy, is your friend. If you look at walking as a teammate in the fight against fat, you more likely will be diligent about your workouts. When you start to look better and feel better, you will know that walking is your friend and partner.

Commitment

Walking for health and weight loss needs firm commitment. Promise yourself that you will work out regularly, and keep your promise. You can make the commitment more concrete by writing up a contract and signing it. You do not need fancy legal terminology for a promise to yourself. You can even go a step further by having the document notarized.

Tell a couple of good friends about your personal promise. Then, if you fail to work out regularly you will feel embarrassed to have to tell them that you are back to a sedentary life. It works best to select two friends who, themselves, exercise regularly. If you have missed a couple of workouts, you will think, "I'd better do a workout this morning so that when I have lunch with Pat and Terry I'll look like I'm in shape. Maybe I'll leave a little sweat on my brow."

Setting and Tending Goals

Setting realistic goals is the *sine qua non* for staying with an exercise program. If your goals are too easily achieved, there will be no challenge or sense of accomplishment. For example, a goal of walking to the newsstand on Saturday night to pick up the Sunday paper is not exactly reaching for the stars. Conversely, a goal that is too difficult will insure failure. Do not expect to walk a marathon two months down the road if you just started a walking program a few weeks ago.

Set long-term goals in general terms and then work on a series of short-term goals one at a time. Instead of setting your sights on 600 miles in a year, aim for three 50-minute workouts this week. When the next week is in sight, plan another three or four workouts. By progressing through such a series of smaller goals, you will get to 600 miles in a year without a year's worth of worrying that you may not achieve your long-term goal.

In setting goals of pace, do not compare yourself to someone else who may be at a different level of fitness. A well-conditioned, veteran walker may need to work out at 5 mph (12 minutes a mile) or better in order to reach a personal aerobic threshold. If you recently started a program of walk training, your aerobic threshold will probably be reached at a pace of about 15 minutes a mile. As you gain experience, your speed will increase, but do not set a deadline for attaining 12 minutes a mile.

Success will come from setting sensible goals and tending to them regularly.

The Means Justify the Means

Attention to the ends—good health and good looks—will contribute to motivational momentum. The means—the actual walking—can be an even stronger motivational force. There are several characteristics that attract us psychologically and physiologically.

o As humans, we are influenced by rhythmic forces. We, ourselves, are a symphony of rhythms: heartbeat, respiration, sleep-wake cycles, sexual rhythms, and many others. Walking with a smooth flow of footsteps adds another rhythm to the score, one that makes us feel like walking on and on.

o Being away from the daily grind and spending time outdoors surrounded by natural light, fresh air, and trees, are additional pleasures of walking.

o   As terrestrial creatures we psychologically need to be in contact with the ground. Walking provides such continuous contact and so adds to mental well being.

o   As we cool down we feel both relaxed and exhilarated.

These qualities of walking are not always on a conscious level. Taking note of them as you walk will give you an appreciation of the process as well as the product. The former—walking—will give you instant gratification. The latter—health—will follow.

Health—Your #1 Priority

Whenever I lecture on aerobic walking, there is invariably someone in the audience who asks whether 20 minutes in the morning and 20 minutes in the evening add up to a single 40-minute workout. It usually turns out that the questioner is walking 20 minutes to work in the morning and 20 minutes home in the evening.

If health and appearance are important to you, then walking deserves its own time and place in your life. Of all life's priorities, health is number one. Walking should be a primary activity, not tacked on to something else for convenience.

Even if your schedule is tight, you can generally make time for three 45-minute workouts a week. The key is to plan ahead. Put each workout on your calendar as an important appointment with an important person—yourself. Write it down, and when someone else makes a request for that time you can honestly say that you are already scheduled.

When you put on your walking shoes, hang a sign on your door that says "In Conference" and head for the park. With a little more self-confidence you can hang a sign that says "Gone Walking."

Larks and Owls

Living on Planet Earth, we are ruled by a 24-hour schedule of light and dark. Many of the chemical reactions of our bodies wax and wane in these circadian rhythms. Our metabolism generally reaches its zenith in the early afternoon, and that is when most of us are most motivated to work out.

Some, however, are at the far sides of the bell curve. The larks among us can be out at 6 AM and be ready to fly at supersonic speed after a minimal warmup. Owls, in contrast, can dance all night and may find late evening hours conducive to a good workout. Whatever your early-late preference, the best time to exercise is when you can schedule your workout or when a free hour appears providentially. The strong rhythms and heightened metabolism of an aerobic workout easily override circadian rhythms. Just get started and go for it.

Sign Up for Walking

Place hand lettered signs around the house to focus your motivation. Here are a few samples for starters:

- o It's easier to exercise for 45 minutes than to be fat for 48 hours.
- o This is a postexercise refrigerator.
- o On your telephone answering machine: I Can Call Back.
- o Over the TV screen: It's a Vast Wasteland, Anyway.

Create a few signs of your own. It's important to change the signs often so they will be visually fresh. Signs can be both fun and a serious behavioral strategy.

Picture Perfect

Signs around the house are a motivational aide, but pictures are even better. Words require reading; pictures hit you right in your feelings. A picture of a grossly fat person and one of a lean, strong athlete can be taped up next to each other. No explanation is needed. Pictures can be placed on critical surfaces: the refrigerator, a full length mirror, the TV set.

Pictures of yourself as you make substantial progress are the best motivators of all. Have someone take photos of you in different outfits and different poses. You can be silly or serious—use your imagination. Fun enhances motivation.

Mind Warming

A good physiological strategy when you are gripped by the blahs is to go out, not for a workout, but for a warmup. Contemplating a full workout when you are not in the mood usually results in sitting down in an easy chair to decide whether or not to do the workout. Invariably, the answer is "Not." Try a five-minute warmup instead and reserve your decision on the workout. The warmup will improve your circulation and raise your spirits. Then it will be easy to go right into the workout and banish the doldrums for the day.

Keeping Records

Keep your walking program in the forefront of your mind by recording each workout in a weekly log (Figure 20). Noting the date and distance (or time) will do the trick. If you would like to add further data such as pace, weather, and mood, so much the better. Personal bests for a given course can be noted in brightly colored ink or with a gold star. Consider adding an occasional whimsical comment:

"No caribou on the trail today."

"Passed a pastry shop but resisted stopping. Good thing it was in the middle of my workout course and not at the end."

"Felt unbelievably strong today. Another few such workouts and I'll be ready to model for the *Sports Illustrated* swimsuit issue."

The log is yours to do with as you wish. Make it a motivational marvel.

Sample Log

Date (day)	Distance	Comments
Friday	45 min.	Worked out right after work—better than beer and small talk at the bar.
Sunday	50 min.	Two joggers got mad when I passed them. I think they were more mad at themselves.
Wednesday	40 min.	Glad to get out of lunch with Jack. Told him I had a prior engagement. I did—with me.

Figure 20.

Event Planning

There is nothing like a special event to give you a sense of purpose in your walking program. Planning to be in a walkathon or to take a long hike to a particular destination will give you a goal.

A few years ago I planned to do a 50-mile walk for peace in Brooklyn's Prospect Park. Until that time I had never walked more than ten continuous miles. I knew the peace walk would take months of training, and so I set aside a few hours each week to get in shape. Starting with three workouts of 4 miles each, I gradually increased the distance of each training session until I reached 10 to 12 miles. In the last month before the big event I put in one workout of 15 miles and one of 18 miles. That event became a powerful motivating force for workouts that were far longer than my usual 45 minutes.

Even if you plan a special event only to motivate yourself, the effect will not be artificial. Add a few frills to the event and you will forget that it was originally a motivational device.

Bribes? Rewards!

There is no shame in setting up a schedule of gifts to reward yourself for greater achievement. For three weeks of regular workouts, you deserve a new T-shirt, headband, or pair of classy socks. Reward yourself every two months with a new warmup suit and every four months with a pair of new walking shoes. The expense is far less than the cost of a therapist or an internist. As for too many exercise outfits, I never knew an athlete who thought it was possible to have too many outfits. I have a clothes closet just for warmup suits, sweatshirts and pants, and sneakers. A dresser drawer is devoted to T-shirts, another to walking shorts, and still another to socks and bandanas. I wear them all.

Your schedule of rewards should be formal and in writing so you can look forward to a day of celebration. Milestone achievements are worth a party with friends. You can wear a new workout outfit that shows off your svelte self.

Watch, Do, Teach

You learn aerobic walking by reading, watching, and receiving instruction. When you have become fairly adept at technique, instruct a poor novice who hardly knows heel from toe. You will be doing a good turn for the new walker and for yourself. Teaching is an incentive to stay in shape so you can be a good role model.

These nineteen ways and means to include exercise in your lifestyle are not a complete list of motivational techniques. You can add anything that works for you. Each of us has a few personal tricks and secrets that provide incentive for action in other spheres of life. Some of them can be effective for exercise.

Do not depend on just one or two strategies to keep your motivation high. Even disciplined people can become weekend warriors, failing to do any workouts at all during the week. Then it is only a short trip to Slothville. Several strategies used at once can work together synergistically to bring you back to regular workouts and the feeling of vitality, good looks, and high health that aerobic walking confers.

CHAPTER 6

The Aerobic Diet Guide for Reducing
The Variety Principle

My co-instructor, Melissa, tells me that she has never seen a dieter who was happy. When Melissa wants to lose a few pounds she works out more and watches her diet only a little. She hardly considers it a diet.

Exercise can obviate the need for dieting, not only by using up calories and improving metabolism, but also by regulating appetite. It is appetite, of course, that gets us into trouble in the first place.

If you are trying to lose weight and have made aerobic walking a regular part of your lifestyle, the *Aerobic Diet Guide for Reducing* will bring you relentless weight loss until you are slim. The *Diet Guide* encourages variety and tasty meals that will keep you from developing an adversarial relationship with your diet. The *Diet Guide* will also lead you to a diet that is rich in nutrients to maintain and even improve your health while you are losing size and weight.

Any reducing diet necessarily reduces total caloric intake, and that reduction limits the quantity of nutrients in the diet. Make the limited number of calories count. Wasting calories on junk food leaves fewer calories in the day's allotment for vitamins and minerals.

Whether dieting or not, the body needs a great range of nutrients for maintaining health. The sources of these nutrients are many and varied among the earth's different foods. Then, it is a matter of preparing the foods well so they will please the palate. These issues are addressed in the three sections of this chapter, *Nutrition Needs, Nutrient Sources,* and *Taste Gains.* The following chapter includes the *Aerobic Diet Guide for Maintenance* and presents the easy transition to the normal, healthful diet that will keep you from returning to your former size and shape.

Nutrient Needs

The intricate and interactive chemistry of the body and brain is supplied by raw materials from the air we breathe and the food we eat. Just as our chemistry is complex, our nutrient needs are extensive.

o The body uses **carbohydrates**—sugars and starches—for the energy of work and play and also for the functioning of the organs that keep us alive.

o The body needs **proteins** for the growth and repair of its tissues.

o The body needs **fats**—in small amounts—for sheaths of nerves and the glands of the skin and endocrine systems.

o The body needs **water** for blood, lymph, cerebrospinal fluid, and the protoplasm of virtually all cells. Most of the chemical reactions of the body take place in a fluid environment that is essentially water-based.

o The body needs **vitamins** and **minerals** for many of its metabolic processes. Countless chemical reactions are turned on and off continually. We need about two dozen vitamins to act as facilitators for these reactions. We need a hundred or so minerals for an even wider variety of basic functions. For example, sodium, potassium, and calcium, individually and in concert, are needed for such diverse work as nerve transmission, kidney function, blood clotting, bone growth, and heart beat regulation.

o The body needs **fiber** and its bulk to stimulate the wave-like contractions of the gastrointestinal tract. These peristaltic contractions move food along for efficient digestion and elimination.

These needs are for both reducing diets and maintenance diets. Let's look at the basics.

Carbohydrates

Carbohydrates are the main energy resource for the body. Every tissue and organ of the body uses blood glucose for its energy needs, and some organs such as the brain rely almost exclusively on glucose. Our total blood glucose supply at any given time is very small, but there is a large reservoir of glucose molecules that the liver holds ready in the form of glycogen. The muscles of the body do not depend solely on blood glucose for their energy but have their own glucose reservoir in the form of muscle glycogen.

When we eat foods with glucose—honey and grape sugar, for instance—the glucose needs no digestion and is quickly absorbed from the gastrointestinal tract. Foods with sucrose—those containing cane or beet sugar—need only one digestive step to split the sucrose molecule into glucose and fructose. In both of these cases, the glucose enters the blood stream quickly and blood sugar levels rise suddenly. In response, the body uses compensatory mechanisms, including the conversion of sugar into fat, to bring the blood glucose level back to normal.

The action guideline for weight loss is to sharply curtail sugar intake. "Sugar" in this context includes: table sugar, honey, maple sugar, and all other sweet syrups, even those made from the conversion of such complex carbohydrates as corn or rice. Any packaged product in which sugar is listed as one of the first few ingredients must be placed on the restricted list. Danger lurks in most of the aisles in the supermarket. Watch out for cereals, canned fruit, crackers, cookies, and such. Always check out the list of ingredients on the labels.

Two foods—perhaps "products" rather than "foods"—that need no checking of labels are chocolate and ice cream. They have a high sugar content as well as a high fat content. To give you an idea of how much sugar is needed to produce the chocolate taste that we are accustomed to, try a bite of the unsweetened chocolate used in baking. Chocolate and ice cream are in the rarest treat category. "Rarest treat" refers to frequency (seldom) and portion size (very small).

Sweets are not totally prohibited. Fruit sugar (fructose) is in a separate metabolic category from glucose, sucrose, and maltose, and only the latter three need avoidance. You actually *should* have three pieces of fruit a day for your reducing diet. A scant amount of fruit puree as a spread on toast—you should still be able to see the surface of the bread—doesn't count as a piece of fruit.

The complex carbohydrates found in grains, starchy vegetables, and legumes must go through a more involved digestive process that takes more time. Such foods do not flood the blood with glucose but, instead, supply energy over a longer period of time without disturbing the balance between blood sugar and lipids. The complex carbohydrates, in fact, enhance stability by providing just enough glucose to keep blood sugar levels between the desired 80 mg and 120 mg.

Proteins

The word *protein* is derived from the Greek *proteios* meaning "first in importance." And so it is—protein is a major part of the structure of every cell, tissue, and organ. Protein is also involved in the synthesis of most enzymes, hormones, and neurotransmitters. We also have maintenance needs for protein because of the constant change in our bodies—the degradation and rebuilding. Approximately one percent to two percent of total body protein turns over each day, and some of that is lost to the body's metabolic processes. The body cannot create protein out of carbohydrates and fats and must rely on dietary protein for replacement.

The average person requires 0.36 grams of protein per pound of body weight (0.8 gram per kg). A 154-pound individual (70 kg) needs 56 grams or 224 calories of protein per day. That recommended daily allowance (RDA) was determined by studying sedentary subjects. You, as a walker, must be considered an endurance athlete with increased protein requirements. Recommendations for an aerobic walker are 0.55 gram per pound per day. That translates to 336 calories worth of protein for the 154-pound person.

Every meal should have some amount of *complete* protein to supply all the essential amino acids necessary for the process of cell and tissue renewal. (See chapter 2 for a list of the essential amino acids.) Omnivores obtain their protein in part from animal sources that supply all the essential amino acids. Vegetarians, in order to

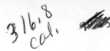
secure all the nutritionally essential amino acids, must employ a strategy of combinations. Legumes and grains, combined, provide such an effective combination. Another way to supply a complete protein from vegetables or grains is to add a small amount of animal proteins.

Fats

Fats are not all bad. They are absolutely essential for many biochemical processes and the integrity of many tissues. But do not worry about having enough total fat in your diet. People, at least in the western world, find that foods with a substantial fat content are tasty. Even an ascetic renouncing the pleasures of the palate gets about ten percent fat in a diet of grains, legumes, and other vegetables.

The type of fat from nonanimal sources such as grains, seeds, nuts, olives, and avocado is mostly monounsaturated fat—a healthful kind. Fish oil contains polyunsaturated omega-3 fats, which also are healthful. Other animal fat sources, including meat, poultry, and dairy products, contain a high concentration of saturated fat—the unhealthful kind. Two *vegetable* sources of saturated fats are palm oil and coconut oil.

In a reducing diet, you must not only avoid saturated fats for health reasons, you must be sparing with all fats.

Water

Our bodies use water and lose water every day. Water is used in a myriad of ways in the metabolic processes of cells, tissues, and organs. Water is lost via the kidneys, bowel, lungs, and skin. We need to replace almost three quarts a day, even if we do not work in a sweat shop. Exercise, naturally, raises the requirements.

We take water in through drinking and eating, and we produce some by oxidation of carbohydrates, fats, and proteins. Most of us drink about a quart of fluid a day. We get another quart from foods that contain a high percentage of water. Another cupful is generated by the oxidation of nutrients. That leaves us almost a quart short of requirements each day. The solution is to have two quarts of noncaffeinated liquid in addition to our food. Extra fluid, beyond daily requirements, is no problem. Our bodies find good use for it in the blood, the lymph, the secretions of the various organs, the fluid between the cells, and the cells themselves. Total body water is substantial, amounting to about 65 percent of the whole body, and an extra quart or so does not create much of a percentage change.

Water intake is important for many reasons: to assure adequate secretions for the digestive tract, to keep the bowel contents soft, to prevent the normal mucous secretions of the respiratory tract from drying out, to keep the blood more fluid for better circulation, and to moisturize the skin from the inside. For those on a weight-loss diet, water is especially important. As fat is metabolized, the organic acids that are formed in the process are excreted more efficiently by the kidneys if there is an accompanying high fluid intake.

The reasons are clear; the prescription is simple. Drink water!

Vitamins

Vitamins were first known for their absence. The deficiency diseases, night blindness, beriberi, scurvy, and rickets, were known long before the idea of vitamins was proposed. At different times in history it was found that butterfat, rice polishings (the part removed to leave nice, white rice), citrus fruits, and cod liver oil, respectively, would cure these diseases. Later, vitamins A, B, C, and D were discovered to be the effective factors.

Biochemistry made strong advances in the beginning of the twentieth century, and a great deal more became known about vitamins. Vitamin B was found to be several vitamins, including thiamine (B1), riboflavin (B2), niacin (sometimes called B3), pyridoxine (B6), cobalamin (B12), pantothenic acid, folic acid, choline, innositol, and biotin. Vitamin K was discovered to be an integral part of the blood clotting mechanism. Vitamin E was found to contribute to reproductive function. The bioflavonoids, associated with vitamin C, were found to prevent capillary fragility.

We now know a great deal more about vitamins, especially their chemistry. Vitamins not only prevent deficiency diseases, they can enhance immune function and slow the aging process of cells and tissues. Vitamins A, C, and E, also serve as antioxidants, comple-

menting the chemicals the body itself produces. The different B vitamins are usually found together in the same food sources and work
together to protect skin, mucous membranes, muscle cells, and
nerves. The vitamins often work hand in hand with mineral elements, as well. Indeed, the body's overall biochemistry is made up of
many interrelated reactions that are in constant coordination in the
service of the entire organism.

Minerals

The body is much like the earth, itself. Both are made up of
over a hundred elements, almost all of which have one or more functions in human physiology. It is generally agreed that even the elements needed in minute amounts and the obscure elements whose
functions are not yet clearly defined are vital to health.

A sampling of minerals whose functions are known will give
you an appreciation of the wide variety of nutrients that the body
and brain need for optimal functioning.

o Sodium, not a devil except in excess, is a key element in regulating acid-base balance, the water rights of the different organs,
electrical conduction along nerves, the formation of digestive
juices, and much of the body's extracellular chemistry.

o Potassium is in continual partial exchange with sodium across
cell membranes, especially in nerve and muscle cells. Potassium
is also a major component of the digestive fluids of the intestines. Recently, in addition to potassium's other functions, it has
been found to be effective in lowering high blood pressure and
in reducing the risk of cerebrovascular stroke.

o Calcium, as every woman knows, is important in preventing osteoporosis. Calcium is also vital for blood clotting, nerve transmission, and muscle contraction of the heart and voluntary muscles.

o Phosphorus, too, is needed for the mineral structure of our
bones, that structure being an intricate form of calcium phosphate. Phosphorus is also an integral part of the high energy
compound A.T.P. (adenosine tri-phosphate) that muscle cells
use for contraction.

o Sulfur is part of the molecular structure of two amino acids—methionine and cysteine—that make up the protein of every cell in our bodies. Sulfur is also a part of many enzymes needed for intermediary metabolism.

o Iron, as we all know, prevents anemia. Iron is the central atom of the hemoglobin molecule that carries oxygen in the red blood cells.

o Magnesium is necessary for the synthesis of proteins and for the contraction of muscle fibers. Magnesium attaches itself to phosphate groups of the high energy compound A.T.P. that is the immediate energy source for that contraction.

o Iodine is used in the structure of thyroid hormone, which takes an active part in energy metabolism.

o Chlorine (as chloride ion) is so ubiquitous in the human body it gets little attention or respect. Yet, it is present in the blood in high concentration and is a necessary ingredient in every body fluid from hydrochloric acid in the stomach to the sweat shed in a hard workout.

o Copper is critical in our lives from birth onward. In infants it is necessary for bone growth and for intellectual development. Throughout life it is needed for iron absorption, protein metabolism, and insuring the strength of blood vessels. Copper is in high concentration in the liver, brain, kidney, and heart—some indication of where it is active. We do not hear much about copper, but it is no penny-ante element. Copper is involved in a wide range of enzymatic/metabolic work that is essential for everyday life.

o Zinc is important in wound healing. There are also some twenty plus enzymes that are zinc-dependent, a sure sign that zinc is basic to many systems of the human organism.

o Manganese functions in a chemically erudite way as a transfer agent in carbohydrate and protein metabolism, and its enzyme chemistry is difficult to reduce to simple terms. For us athlete-walkers, the bottom line is that manganese is important to the integrity of our tendons and bones. Manganese also takes part in antioxidant activity, which keeps our tissues young.

o Selenium is integral to one of the body's natural antioxidants—glutathione peroxidase. Selenium and vitamin E, are synergistic, each enhancing the effect of the other in their antioxidant activity.

o Molybdenum does not trip lightly on the tongue. It is as heavy in its chemistry as in its syllables. Its metabolism is not well understood, but it is known to participate in different oxidase systems.

o Chromium as an earthly element is familiar to us all, thanks to the steel industry. Our bodies, of course, recognized the need for chromium long before the advent of chrome plated Buick grills. Chromium, acting in concert with insulin, is necessary for glucose metabolism. Chromium interacts with other metabolic cycles: it must cooperate with iron, it may compete with zinc, and it helps to regulate lipoproteins.

o Silicon is involved in connective tissue metabolism. It plays a role in the synthesis of collagen fibers throughout our bodies. The result is firm, supple skin and strong, resilient ligaments and tendons. Beautiful athletes need dietary silicon.

o Vanadium moderates lipid metabolism, inhibiting the synthesis of cholesterol and reducing triglycerides. It is also important for the development of bone, showing up in high concentrations where mineralization is active. Another function is in reproduction. Animal studies have shown higher survival rates in the newborn whose mothers had optimum vanadium levels.

o This space is reserved for other trace elements, often needed in extremely small amounts and whose function may not yet be fully known.

Dietary Fiber

This last dietary factor is not a nutrient; yet, it is necessary in our diets. Fiber stimulates peristalsis, the intestines' slow, wave-like contractions that move everything along. Adequate fiber helps to normalize gastrointestinal function. In the stomach and the duodenum (the first part of the small intestine), fiber bulk promotes satiety. In the large intestine, fiber absorbs water and adds to volume. It prevents diarrhea as well as constipation. Overall, fiber-rich foods shorten total transit time through the digestive tract and so lessen the amount of time that potentially carcinogenic substances excreted by the liver are in contact with the colon.

Fiber, itself, is not a single entity and, as such, is found in many diverse kinds of foods. Some types of fiber are water soluble, and others are not. Several varieties of fiber occur commonly in foods. Because the different types of fiber work in somewhat different ways, it is best to have a variety of fiber sources in your diet. Avoid refined foods; they have much of their fiber removed in the processing.

Nutrient Sources

The body's nutrient needs are many, varied, and complex. Supplying all the nutrients in their proper proportions seems like an almost impossible mission. If we tried to meet the needs one by one, it surely would be impossible. A little insight, however, makes the task less daunting.

We know that the foods we eat are grown in the earth or derived from it. The earth (including the sea) and its plant and animal life contain everything our bodies require, each food source providing not one but several nutrients. It makes eminent sense to depend on nature rather than on manufactured supplements as the principal source of the 100+ nutrients our bodies must have for health. The widest variety of foods, naturally, supply the widest variety of nutrients.

Beyond variety, my new "Eight-Category Family of Foods" (Figure 21) provides more specific guidelines for food selection. It will lead to a diet with a balanced supply of all the vital nutrients. The Family of Foods is the framework for both the *Aerobic Diet Guide for Reducing* and the *Aerobic Diet Guide for Maintenance*.

Eight-Category Family of Foods

1. Salad vegetables—generous
2. Green and yellow vegetables—generous
3. Grains—generous
4. Fruits—moderate to generous
5. Starchy vegetables—moderate
6. Legumes—moderate
7. Dairy—moderate, if low fat; sparing, if made with whole milk
8. Animal proteins—sparing

Definitions: Generous, Moderate, Sparing

The foods that are to be used most generously are at the top of the list, and those that should be used sparingly are at the bottom.

Generous means a nice-sized portion (but not extra large) at every meal. A nice-sized portion fits on a $9^1/_2$-inch dinner plate without overlapping the edges and without covering 98 percent of the surface.

Moderate means a nice portion at one meal or, alternately, a moderate portion at one meal and a small portion at another meal during the day. A moderate portion fits comfortably on an 8-inch plate. A small portion fits on a $6^1/_2$-inch plate without crowding the edges.

Sparing means a small portion at one meal a day.

Figure 21.

General Rules for Using
the Family of Foods Chart

The sources of each of the nutrients that our bodies need are always found in more than one food and usually in more than one of the eight categories. Some foods may be properly placed in more than one category. For example, spinach can be a salad vegetable or a green vegetable. Bean sprouts are part legume and part salad vegetable. Corn can be a grain or a yellow vegetable.

The Family of Foods, thus, is somewhat flexible as a guide. Be fair when following the advice on portion size and frequency, and do not overdo any one food. You will find it easy to become healthy and lean.

Salad Vegetables

✓celery	✓Jerusalem artichoke	✓scallions
✓cucumber	✓lettuce	✓snow peas
dandelion greens	✓mushrooms	✓spinach
endive	✓parsley	sprouts
escarole	✓peppers (green and red)	✓tomatoes
fennel	radishes	watercress

Salad vegetables usually are eaten raw, although some of them can also be cooked. Served raw, the leafy vegetables occupy a large amount of space on the plate. Thus, a serving that is visually ample is very low in calories, in good part because a serving does not weigh much. The total amount of nutrition in a light-weight serving also is low. But these are good reasons to be generous with salads.

Salad vegetables provide some vitamins and minerals and are a good source of fiber. The less-known B vitamins—choline, folic acid, and PABA—are present in leafy green vegetables. Leafy greens also supply calcium, cobalt, and vitamin K. Spinach and dandelion greens are rich in vitamin A, parsley offers vitamin C, and tomatoes and red and green peppers contain both vitamins A and C. These are only a few examples of individual nutrients present in individual salad vegetables. Many other nutrients in smaller amounts are also supplied by the salad vegetable group.

Some nutritionists are concerned that lettuce, spinach, and other salad vegetables are eaten raw. Washing them with water may remove the dirt and sand but not bacteria and parasites. One solution that has been recommended is to make up a disinfectant solution of two tablespoons of vinegar per quart of water and let the vegetables soak for a half hour. The idea has merit.

While salad vegetables are a good source for many nutrients, you cannot depend on this group alone for all your nutritional needs. Keep salads in perspective.

Green and Yellow Vegetables

artichokes	carrots	kale
asparagus	cauliflower	rhubarb
beets	collards	spinach
beet greens	corn	summer squash
broccoli	eggplant	Swiss chard
Brussels sprouts	green beans	turnips
cabbage	green peas	zucchini

Green and yellow vegetables are obtained from the seeds, fruits, pods, flowers, stems, roots, or leaves of particular plants. These vegetables generally are cooked, though a few of them can also be eaten raw. These vegetables, with two exceptions, are low in calories, and you can afford to be liberal in your servings. The two exceptions are corn and green peas, both of which are calorically moderate. Serve the exceptions in moderate amounts, and be generous with the rest.

This category, rich in many nutrients, is a vital part of any healthful diet. These vegetables contribute a modest amount of complex carbohydrates and substantial amounts of many vitamins and minerals. Broccoli, kale, asparagus, and collards are rich in the B vitamin, riboflavin. Cabbage contributes another of the B vitamins, pyridoxine. Carrots supply vitamin A in the form of beta carotene, and cauliflower contains vitamin K. Kale and broccoli also provide calcium, and spinach supplies iron. Each vegetable of the group contains several nutrients, but in each case it is a different several. It is wise to include a wide variety from this category in your diet.

Green and yellow vegetables, while being high in nutrients, are low in fat and in calories and so make the perfect centerpiece for a reducing diet.

Grains

Cereal Grasses		Noncereal Grass Plants
wheat	rye	buckwheat
rice	barley	amaranth
oats	millet	quinoa
corn		

Grain-Containing Foods
bread, muffins, rolls, bagels, biscuits, pita, pizza
crackers, flatbread, pretzels
pancakes, waffles
breakfast cereal
stuffings
rice dishes
pasta and noodles (wheat, buckwheat, or rice)
soups containing grains (barley, corn, rice, etc.)
granola (oats and other grains)
couscous (usually wheat)
kasha (buckwheat)
pilafs
risoto (rice)
hominy (corn)

Grains are a rich source of many nutrients, yet are not highly caloric. They deserve a "generous" rating in your diet. Certain high-calorie foods that are often used with grains—such as butter, cheese, and oils—must be minimized in a reducing diet.

Grains are a great source of complex carbohydrates, which are the body's preferred energy source for both daily activities and sports and exercise.

The cereal grass grains supply many of the amino acid building blocks of protein, but are deficient in one or more of the *essential* amino acids, most often lysine. The missing amino acids can be obtained from legumes, the noncereal grass grains buckwheat and amaranth, and animal sources.

Grains are fairly low in fat content and, unless they have been made into doughnuts or fettucine Alfredo, will not sabotage your low-fat diet intentions.

Grains are a good source of many vitamins and minerals. All the vitamins of the B complex group except for B12 are richly supplied by whole grain foods. B12, not found in any plant source, must be obtained from animal-derived foods or laboratory-made supplements. Whole grains also supply vitamin E. The minerals iron, magnesium, manganese, chromium, selenium, silicon, and phosphorus are found in moderate to high levels in the grains. Zinc is also found abundantly in the grains, but our digestive systems cannot extract it easily. Zinc is better absorbed from meat, eggs, and seafood.

Whole grains, including the outer bran layer, are a fine source of fiber. The bran of different grains contains different types of fiber, a good reason for including a variety of grains in your diet.

Fruits

apples ✓	figs ✓	papayas ✓
apricots ✓	grapes ✓	peaches ✓
bananas ✓	guavas	pears ✓
berries ✓	kiwis ✓	persimmons
cherries ✓	lychees	pineapples ✓
citrus fruits ✓	mangoes	plums ✓
currants	melons ✓	pomegranates
dates ✓	nectarines ✓	

The category of fruits is extensive with great variety. Fruits vary in size from tiny wild cranberries to huge watermelons. Each fruit has a distinctive taste, most with an underlying sweetness and a few with added tartness. A chef could not wish for more choices.

For all their differences, fruits contain a high percentage of the sugar fructose. An exception is grapes, whose main sugar is glucose. Fructose, though a simple sugar, is not quickly absorbed from the small intestine or rushed into the blood stream by the liver. Thus, it acts more like a complex carbohydrate.

Fruits, in addition to supplying carbohydrates, are filled with vitamins and minerals. Fruits with an orange color are generally rich in vitamin A. Mangoes, papayas, apricots, and cantaloupes are especially good sources. Vitamin C is found in many fruits, but especially in strawberries, oranges, lemons, and papayas. Bioflavonoids, needed for the integrity of connective tissues and capillaries, are found in the same fruits that have vitamin C and are found in particularly high amounts in black currants, cherries, and oranges. The B vitamins are present in most fruits in moderate amounts. Fruits, though not as good a source of the B complex group as grains, do contribute significant amounts of these vitamins to any diet.

Minerals vary a great deal from fruit to fruit. Mangoes supply surprisingly high quantities of iron. Blueberries and blackberries also furnish iron. Oranges and bananas are good sources of potassium. Raisins contain copper. Cobalt is found in several different fruits. The path to as many vitamins and minerals as possible is variety.

Many fruits are a good source of fiber. The best are apples, figs, plums, pineapple, apricots, and cherries. Fruit juice that does not contain the pulp of the fruit is essentially devoid of fiber.

The fruits category, at first glance, seems like wonderfood— nutritious and delightful to the taste. But fruits require a little caution. The fructose and fiber content of fruit, if ingested in large amounts, causes diarrhea and consequent *loss* of nutrients. Be careful, too, with most dried fruits. They are higher in calories by weight than the same fresh fruit. Dates are a particular culprit in raising the calorie count.

Overall, fruits should be moderate to generous in a reducing diet. Three servings a day is just about right.

Starchy Vegetables

breadfruit	sweet potatoes and yams
lima beans ✓	potatoes
parsnips	pumpkin
plantain	winter squash (all varieties)

Potato, the starchy vegetable of choice of the majority of Americans, is not necessarily a "fattening" food. Baked potato laden with sour cream, mashed potatoes smothered with butter, and potato strips that are deep fried are all fattening, but not for their potato content. The starchy vegetables in this category are low in fat and high in complex carbohydrates. They also contain a small but significant amount of protein.

The different starchy vegetables contain different vitamins and minerals. White potatoes have a fair amount of the B vitamins and only a trace of vitamin A. Sweet potatoes are low in the B vitamins and rich in vitamin A. Parsnips are low in niacin and high in riboflavin and thiamine, among the B complex vitamins. The minerals vary from one starchy vegetable to another and even from farm to farm where they are grown—all the more reason to include a variety of starchy vegetables in the diet.

One attribute that all the vegetables in this category share is fiber. Winter squash, parsnips, and pumpkin are especially good sources.

Legumes

adzuki beans	kidney beans
black eyed peas	lentils
black turtle beans	mung beans
cranberry beans	navy beans
fava beans	pinto beans
green pigeon beans	soy beans (tofu)
split peas	

Legumes serve multiple nutritional needs. They supply both carbohydrate and protein, yet little fat. The carbohydrate is complex and does not upset the body's energy balance. The protein contains most of the essential amino acids, but is low in methionine. Grains and legumes, thus, complement each other to for a complete protein.

Legumes are a good source of most of the B vitamins, with the notable exception of B12. As with grains you must supplement the other B vitamins of legumes with B12 from animal or laboratory sources. Legumes also provide many minerals, including: calcium, copper, manganese, phosphorus, and potassium. Tofu is especially high in calcium because it is made into solid form by coagulating soymilk with calcium compounds.

Legumes are a good source of fiber, a final reason for including this category of foods in a balanced diet.

All the nutritional reasons for including legumes in the diet must be tempered with their moderate caloric content. Legumes are best combined with foods from other categories.

Dairy Products

Dairy products supply calcium (the good news) and saturated fat (the bad news). There are many other pieces of good news and a few bulletins of bad news.

Dairy foods are a source of all the essential amino acids; two or more essential fatty acids; enzyme proteins; generous amounts of vitamins A, D, and K; most of the B vitamins including B12 and the lesser known ones such as lecithin, cephalin, folic acid, and choline; and the minerals, potassium, magnesium cobalt, and phosphorus.

Further good news comes in the form of yogurt, which contains active Lactobaccilus cultures. These cultures protect the health of mucous membranes, especially the gastrointestinal and genito-urinary tracts. The bacteria also predigest a good part of the lactose in the yogurt—good news for lactose-intolerant individuals. And, the lactic acid that is produced aids the absorption of calcium.

The good news in the dairy case must be balanced with further bad news: most milk is homogenized before sending it to market. Homogenization breaks up the fat globules into such small droplets that they can be absorbed from the small intestine before they are completely digested. This overburdens the liver and makes the blood a little milky for a while. The solution is to buy nonfat milk or non-homogenized low-fat milk. The last of the bad news is that milkfat, which contains a high percentage of saturated fat, is not only athero-genic, it is highly caloric. Sweet cream, sour cream, and hard cheeses are the worst offenders. Milk, cottage and other soft cheeses, and yogurt are made in low-fat varieties. Dairy products made from skim milk or, one percent low-fat milk at most, contain most of the nutrients but are low in fat and moderate in calories. Use these low-fat and nonfat dairy products in moderate amounts. Nonfat yogurt, with its general and special health gifts, can be a star in your reducing diet.

Animal Proteins

Meat, poultry, eggs, and seafood, all of which come from animal sources, supply protein that contains a complete set of amino acids. It is higher grade protein than is found in plant sources. In addition, animal protein foods contain generous amounts of many other nutrients. But there are significant problems with animal sources of protein. Let's take meat, poultry, eggs, and seafood and examine the positives and negatives one category at a time.

Meats contain an abundance of B complex vitamins, including B12. Organ meats contain vitamin E. Liver contains vitamins A, E, and K. Meats also supply a large variety of minerals including potassium, phosphorus, zinc, iron, copper, and calcium.

As rich as meat is in these nutrients, so is it rich in fat—saturated fat, at that. The effect of dietary fat on size and weight and the effect of saturated fat on health are well known.

Another negative factor is that livestock herds are often treated with antibiotics and sometimes with hormones. Even very small "acceptable" residues cannot be healthy. Meats should be used sparingly in a diet and the fat should be trimmed off. Meat should be used more as a complement to main dishes of grains and vegetables, rather than as an entree.

Poultry contains many of the same nutrients as meat, though vitamins and minerals are often more abundant in meats. An advantage of chicken and turkey is that most of the fat is right under the skin and can be removed with the skin. The negative side of poultry is that chickens, like steer, are often given antibiotics. In addition, the birds' living conditions on many farms are less than sanitary and many chickens come to market carrying pathogenic bacteria. Preparing and cooking chicken must be done with care.

Poultry, like meat, is best used to complement grains and vegetables.

Eggs have gotten especially bad press because they contain the highest level of cholesterol of any food, but eggs are not the sole culprit when cholesterol is too high. Total fat intake is even more to blame. Our bodies easily manufacture cholesterol from dietary fats. There also are differences from one person to another. Some individuals can eat several eggs a week and show no effect. Others are more sensitive to dietary cholesterol.

Eggs have nutritionally redeeming features that make them worth including in modest amounts in a healthful diet. Eggs contain protein that is well balanced in essential amino acids. Eggs contain phosphorus, calcium, magnesium, potassium, sulfur, and iron. Eggs are rich in vitamin A and in many of the B complex vitamins.

You need not give up eggs entirely; just be sparing. A good rule of thumb is: no more than two or three eggs a week, one at a sitting.

Seafood ought to be a superfood. Fish and shellfish, in addition to their complete protein, contain a variety of vitamins and minerals and a modest amount of unsaturated fat of the kind that supplies essential fatty acids. But in recent years, lakes and seas have become polluted with many kinds of toxic chemicals and the life forms of the world's waters have become contaminated to a greater or lesser extent. Closed and semiclosed bodies of water that have industrial plants along their shores are highly suspect. Where currents and tides regularly bring in water from the open ocean, there is less danger. An educated guess is that seafood twice a week would represent a good balance of substantial benefit and minimal harm.

Taste Gains

An adversarial relationship with a weight-loss diet usually results in failure. Conversely, a diet that offers variety and is pleasing to the palate makes long-term success a likelihood.

There are many tricks of the kitchen trade to make vegetables, grains, and fruit into tasty dishes. Many of these are palate principles rather than recipes, and the recipes that are included here are fairly simple. Preparing a healthful, tasty menu does not require esoteric equipment. Pots, pans, baking dishes, a steamer, and a blender or food processor are the basics.

Let's check the Family of Foods categories and sample some seasonings, dressings, sauces, and toppings that make for a tasteful diet. Let's combine foods whose flavors are complementary. Then, let's look after snacks, an important part of daily life. Finally there are trade-ins for fats, sweets, meats, and eggs.

Salad Vegetables

Any selections from the salad veggie list can be combined to suit any fancy. Mushrooms go well with fresh spinach leaves. Sliced radishes add color and a little tang. Fennel provides a licorice-fresh taste. Sprouts from any seeds or beans—not just alfalfa—contribute variety. Sprouts of pumpkin seeds (pepitas) add a nice bitter touch. My favorite crunchy ingredient is thinly-sliced Jerusalem artichokes.

The danger zone in salads starts at the dressings. Fat has been the primary ingredient in salad dressings since lettuce and olives were first cultivated in the ancient world. Oil, even if it is monounsaturated and healthful, contains 9 calories per gram or over 100 calories per tablespoon. But you can create your own dressings, using no oil at all. The following recipes each add an individualistic taste to salads at a small cost in calories.

Basic White Salad Dressing
$\frac{1}{2}$ cup plain yogurt (nonfat)
1 tsp. lemon juice
$\frac{1}{2}$ tsp. dill
2 turns ground pepper
  Use 2 tbs. per serving
  Yield: $4\frac{1}{2}$ servings

Red Dressing
$\frac{1}{2}$ cup tomato juice
1 clove minced garlic
1 tsp. chopped fresh basil
1 tbs. lime or lemon juice
1 small scallion, minced
2 turns ground pepper
  Use 2 tbs. per serving
  Yield: 5 servings

Hot Is Cool
$\frac{1}{2}$ cup plain yogurt (nonfat)
$\frac{1}{2}$ tsp. white horseradish
$\frac{1}{4}$ tsp. basil
$\frac{1}{4}$ tsp. dill
  Use 2 tbs. per serving
  Yield: 4 servings

The serving size is listed for each of these recipes to keep you honest in your perception of an adequate amount of dressing for a salad. I have seen some overly generous perceptions of "adequate" during my many weekends at the health spa where I teach aerobic walking. Their salad bar has three canisters, each with a different low-calorie salad dressing. The canisters are supplied with 4-table-spoon ladles. Every time I have been there I have seen two or three large guests fill their plates, then saturate the salad with two ladles of low-calorie dressing. If and when such individuals do lose weight, how will they maintain the lower weight when they return to a reg-ular diet? It is much better to establish good perceptions and atti-tudes while you are reducing; then you will be a long-term success.

Green and Yellow Vegetables

Most of the vegetables in this category really are green or yel-low; a few are red or white. All can use at least a little cooking. Even carrots, which are sometimes eaten raw, are more digestible when steamed for five minutes. Most vegetables in this category can be steamed or stir fried, and a few can be baked. For those vegetables that become tender quickly—such as zucchini and broccoli tops—steaming is the best method.

The green and yellow vegetables have individual needs for fla-vor enhancement. Here are a few ideas for addings and toppings.

o Grated Romano or Parmesan cheese goes well on zucchini, broccoli, and cauliflower. Two teaspoonsful weigh less than ¼ ounce but are packed with flavor.

o Add 2 tsp. lime juice to steamed Swiss chard and sprinkle with toasted sesame seeds. Serve whole grain crackers or flatbread on the side.

o Sliver almonds and add to steamed green beans. Grind on a little black pepper.

o Add diced red and green pepper to corn.

o Cabbage and Brussels sprouts can use a couple of dashes of lemon juice. A sprinkle of caraway seeds adds a little zip.

o A sprinkling of grated nutmeg makes carrots special.

Green vegetables must not be steamed too long. These vegetables should retain their bright green color. Crisp tastes better.

Most of the vegetables in the green and yellow category may also be marinated after they are blanched. Lemon juice, or equal parts of lemon juice and wine vinegar, with added salt, pepper, and herbs makes an effective oil-free marinade. Allow the vegetables to marinate for two hours or more in the refrigerator, and then serve as a cold antipasto with two slices of crusty French bread.

Grains

The grains list in the previous section offers an idea of the many ways to use the various grains in your diet. A variety of the different cereal grass and noncereal grass grains delivers a variety of nutrients. The different forms in which these grains are processed and prepared keeps your diet interesting as you lose size and weight.

Grains are commonly ground into flour for baking. Wheat flour is so common it is called all-purpose flour. Flour is also made from rye, oats, amaranth, quinoa, and the other grains. The noncereal grass grains—buckwheat, amaranth, and quinoa—make fine hot cereals and pancakes, can substitute for rice in casseroles and other rice dishes, and may be used as flour in multigrain breads, muffins, and (yum) popovers. Cornmeal, though not quite a flour, is tasty as corn muffins and corn bread. I have even heard of cornmeal pizza crust.

Wheat comes in different varieties and forms. Flour, of course, is used for bread and cake, and durum wheat semolina for pasta. Whole wheat flour requires a little experience to handle well. A good suggestion is to start with whole wheat pancakes rather than whole wheat bread. After that you can try dealing with proofing yeast and kneading dough. Then you can use sourdough starter instead of yeast.

Wheatberries and bulgur can be used as the grain itself without grinding, flaking, or otherwise processing. They require only boiling in water. Wheatberries take an hour if they are first soaked overnight; bulgur takes 15 minutes without presoaking. Couscous, which is a kind of pasta in tiny pebbled form, takes only 5 minutes in boiling water. All three can be used with vegetables in casseroles and in soups.

Rice is the staff of life for most of the world's population. It comes in several varieties and is used in untold numbers of recipes with chicken, fish, legumes, and vegetables, as well as in soups and puddings.

For health, it is best to use whole (or brown) rice. Brown rice, if cooked properly, does not come out sticky. The trick is to avoid overcooking it. I prefer the long grain variety and use 1 cup of rice to $1^{3}/_{4}$ cups of water. Rinse the rice and place in a heavyweight pot of boiling water. Cover the pot tightly, return to a boil momentarily, and then reduce heat to a minimum and allow to simmer. Total cooking time is 40 to 45 minutes. Uncover the pot and, as the rice cools, mix a couple of times with a wooden spoon so the bottom layer doesn't continue to cook while the pot is still hot. Instant white rice may be quicker, but the brown rice does not need attention while it is simmering.

This simple boiled rice can be the basis of an entire meal. Just add a legume, diced tomato, zucchini or broccoli, a sprinkling of olive oil, and a dash of tamari. A little basil (or any other herb) and a couple of turns of ground pepper add a finishing touch. You can use other vegetables such as diced green or red pepper or sliced olives. Make your own recipes to please your own palate.

Oats are not only the little flattened flakes we know as rolled oats. In Scotland, oats are usually steel-cut, which produces sliced rather than flattened grain. Steel-cut oats are available in the United States and are cooked just like rolled oats. It takes longer but results in a grainier texture and better taste.

Barley is not just for making soup or beer. Boil barley as you would rice, add steamed or sauteed vegetables, season, and you have a tasty pilaf-equivalent.

Millet grows as small, round, yellow-to-orange seeds. It cooks in less time than rice, about 25 minutes, and can be used in soups and in baked goods.

Rye once was used in several forms: rye berries, cracked rye, and rye flour. Today it is used mostly as flour for bread. Rye breads have a hearty aroma and flavor, distinctive enough not to be overwhelmed by caraway, anise, or grated orange peel. A quick search of cookbooks comes up with recipes for Swedish rye bread, sourdough rye, a couple of Scandinavian flatbreads, rye beer bread, and even rye-and-caraway pancakes.

Rye is still available as rye berries (kernels) and cracked rye, though you may have to search for them. In these forms it can be used as a cooked breakfast cereal, for soups, and in the other ways that wheat is used. With rye, it is not variety for variety's sake alone. It is adding taste with a little zing.

The cultivation of grain was responsible, in good part, for the rise of civilization. When families of hunter-gatherers learned to plant grain, they could establish homesites. The early farms and villages had limited choices of grains—barley in the Near East and millet in the Far East. You can count yourself lucky to have so many choices among today's grains. Enjoy a variety from Category 3 in the Family of Foods, and be generous in the total number of servings each day.

Fruits

Fruits have a pleasant, sweet taste. In addition to sweetness, each fruit has its own taste, distinct from every other. The full range is as wide as any chef could wish for.

The category of fruits is extensive, and the recipes and ways of serving fruit are many. Fruits are generally tasty enough to serve just as they come from the tree or vine. They also can also be made into salads, soups, sauces, compotes, and so forth. Fruit can be baked, poached, or used to flavor and highlight other foods.

Most fruit dishes need no sweetening. In fact, fruit juice can be used as a sweetening in other recipes. Apple, grape, and orange juices are the usual heroes in keeping sugar to a minimum.

A potpourri of helpful hints and suggestions will get you started in making fruit a regular part of your diet.

Applesauce is one of the basics. It is so basic, the word *applesauce* is one word instead of two. The product sold in the supermarket tastes factory-made (which it is). You can produce much better applesauce in your own kitchen. The following basic recipe will result in an uncommonly tasty dish.

Applesauce
6 tart apples
½ lemon, sliced thinly
¼ cup water
¼ cup apple juice
1 stick cinnamon
2 tbs. raisins
1 tbs. maple syrup
  (or honey)

Cut, core, peel, and slice each apple into water containing a little lemon juice. That keeps the apples from turning brown during preparation. Place the apple slices, lemon slices, and cinnamon stick into a sauce pan with the water and apple juice. Bring the covered pan to a boil, then simmer for 9 to 10 minutes until the apples are almost tender. Add raisins and maple syrup, and simmer another two minutes. Mash with a potato masher to the consistency you like. For me, lumpy applesauce is best. Serve with a dollop of yogurt on top.

Baked apples are more elegant than applesauce and easier to prepare. Select tart apples such as Greenings or Granny Smiths. Core the apples, score through the skin with longitudinal lines (from north to south), and place in a small oven-proof bowl. Fill the core hole halfway with raisins, one level teaspoonful, and bake at 350° for about 20 minutes until the score lines widen and the apple is tender. Be careful not to overcook. Drip a teaspoonful of maple syrup on top of each apple and serve.

Dried fruit invites eating right out of the package. Be wary: It can become a mindless habit. Dried fruit is smaller in size than the fresh fruit it once was. You will not realize you are eating much until you think in terms of the fresh fruit equivalent. A handful of raisins, for example, is about the same as a full bunch of grapes. Measure dried fruit as if it were fresh. Dates and figs, which are fairly caloric, can be kept under control by cubing or chopping one or two of them and adding the many small pieces to yogurt or fruit salad. Reserve dried fruit for a special treat, not a twice-a-day snack right out of the package.

For compote, use either fresh or dried fruit. Choose any combination of peaches, pears, prunes, apricots, and a few raisins. Add a few strips of lemon peel and enough water to cover the bottom of the saucepan to ¾ inch. Simmer with the pan covered until everything is tender. Dried fruit takes about 20 minutes; fresh fruit takes about a third less time. Allowing the compote to remain covered on a pilot light for additional time continues the process and results in a richer syrup for the fruit. The compote goes well on a dish of plain yogurt. For that matter, yogurt goes well on a dessert cup of compote. You can also puree a portion of the compote in a blender to make wonderful jam.

Another variety of fruit puree is made by simmering blueberries (either fresh or frozen) in enough water to cover for about 30 minutes and mashing them with a potato masher every so often. The puree thickens as it cools. It is as simple as that.

Fresh fruit salad is a matter of cutting up whatever fruit you like and tossing it with two tablespoons of buttermilk enhanced with grated nutmeg.

These few ideas should get you started on checking out other fruit recipes. Avoid those that use more than a minimum of sugar, honey, or syrup. Of course, nature's own recipe is plain, ripe fruit straight from the vine or tree.

Starchy Vegetables

Here are a few ways to dress up these vegetables to please the palate:

o Boiled red potatoes can be made appealing by leaving the skins on, cutting them in eighths, and topping with finely chopped parsley. An alternative to parsley is rosemary.

o Baked potatoes can be enhanced with low-fat (or no-fat) yogurt. Mixing the yogurt one-to-one with low-fat cottage cheese makes it pretty close to sour cream in taste and consistency. Do not overwhelm the potato with the dressing—two teaspoonsful is generous enough.

o Winter squash can be baked whole, cut in half, and served with two teaspoonsful of maple syrup. One variety, buttercup squash, is somewhat sweet in itself and may need only one teaspoonful of syrup.

o Spaghetti squash is special for its texture. Bake it whole, cut it in half, remove the seeds, score the flesh with a fork, and scoop it from its shell with a spoon. This stringy vegetable can be served hot or cold with halved cherry tomatoes, diced green pepper, minced garlic, and a sprinkle of olive oil and wine vinegar.

o Parsnips are not just a soup ingredient. They can stand on their own if prepared as follows: Slice, cube, steam for ten minutes, and then puree the cooked parsnips in a blender with aliquots of low-fat milk until they come out looking like whipped potatoes. Add some grated nutmeg, and, *voila*, you have a slightly sweet vegetable with a distinctive taste.

o Plantains are nutritionally in the category of a starchy vegetable, but they become sweet if you allow them to over-ripen until they are black-skinned and fairly soft to the touch. Cut off the ends and score through the skin lengthwise on four sides with the tip of a paring knife. Bake for about 20 minutes at 350°. Peel and serve with a teaspoonful of honey or maple syrup per plantain.

Legumes

The category of legumes includes more than just beans. Legumes come in dozens of varieties and are used by almost all cultures around the world. The legume list contains a fair variety, but there are surely others that can be added.

Beans have been the source of no end of jokes. Mel Brooks' *Blazing Saddles* owes at least a part of its success to the lowly bean and its mischievous skills. But, there is a way out of the embarrassment—beans can be degasified.

The U.S.D.A. has researched the problem and they advise: Boil the beans in a large amount of water (5 cups of water per cup of beans) for 10 minutes. Let cool overnight, discard the water, and then cook until done. The time for cooking depends on the variety of bean and how firm or soft you prefer your beans, but one to several hours is generally needed.

Other authorities have suggested discarding the water two or three times during cooking and using a splash of vinegar at least once. Some chefs say that including citrus fruit in the same meal reduces the gas from beans. It also makes sense to eat a small quantity of beans at two meals rather than a large serving at one meal. And, eat slowly. Having good digestion shortens the transit time of intestinal contents. That leaves less time for the bacteria to produce gas. Regular exercise, of course, helps digestion.

Now that that problem is solved, we can concentrate on the desirable qualities of the lowly bean. Legumes can enhance a meal with not only nutrients but also texture, color, and taste.

Legumes can be added to vegetable salads, casseroles, and soups. The legumes should be firm for salads, soft for soups, and in between for casseroles.

Beans, once cooked, can also be marinated for a couple of hours, or even overnight, and used as part of an antipasto offering along with marinated mushrooms, cauliflower, artichoke hearts, and/or beets. The marinade can be as simple as a wine vinegar to which you add basil or other herbs and a turn of freshly ground pepper. You may add a few slices of garlic to flavor the marinade further.

Beans are a substantial part of chili recipes. Chili is versatile and can be served on rice or noodles or with whole grain bread. Chili recipes can be made cooler by reducing the chili pepper content. Paprika is not hot except in appearance and can replace some of the hot peppers. Cumin, also not hot, gives the dish a Mexican flavor. Tailor the recipe to your own taste.

Lentil-vegetable soups are hearty and nutritious. Substituting dry white wine for part of the water in the recipe will add a zesty taste, even after the alcohol has evaporated.

Split pea soup is a perennial favorite. If made to a stick-to-the-ribs consistency and eaten with a whole grain bread, it is a meal in itself.

Lentils and split peas need no soaking and cook in much less time than beans. Pink lentils need eight to ten minutes—practically no time at all as compared to other legumes. If prepared with wine in the recipe, there may be a little alcohol left when served.

Little adzuki beans, a quarter inch in length, can be used in a recipe that I call "Sunrise Surprise." Add cooked adzuki beans to mandarin orange sections and dress with a mixture of 1 tsp. vegetable oil, $\frac{1}{2}$ tsp. wine vinegar, and a touch of prepared mustard. The dish is served cold and is appropriate any time of day. Adzuki beans are the most digestible of all beans and can be used generously in the recipe.

Tofu, a soy bean curd, comes in several forms and can be used in many recipes. Simply slice firm tofu into cubes and add them to a salad. You might take it a step further by adding a sprinkle of sesame seeds and a brief dash of tamari or shoyu, the traditional Chinese or Japanese fermented soy sauces. The softer "silken" tofu (my own favorite) can be substituted for the firm variety.

Dozens and dozens of recipes have been devised using tofu as the main ingredient—everything from tofu burgers to strawberry tofu dessert. Tofu can also be pan fried and dressed with special sauce. Here is Melissa's recipe:

Special Sauce for Tofu
1 part lemon juice
1 part apple cider
1 part tamari
sprinkling of sesame seeds
sliced scallion
few dashes of Worcestershire sauce
1 dash Tabasco sauce
Mix ingredients together.

To make pan-fried tofu, use a seasoned cast iron (or nonstick) pan, wipe with the few drops of sesame oil, heat, and move the cubes of tofu around for the first minute to prevent sticking. Repeat on four sides of the cubes. Serve hot and spoon sauce onto cubes of tofu.

Tofu is a fine protein source, soy beans being the closest of all legumes to providing a complete protein. The soy bean also extracts many valuable mineral elements from the soil. Unfortunately, soy beans are not discriminating and may extract aluminum as well as potassium, calcium, phosphorus, and iron. Do not overdo the tofu.

Legumes and grains form a complete protein and can be the basis of a main dish. Thus, any legume with any cereal grass grain has all the essential amino acids. A good example is pasta salad that includes legumes as well as other vegetables.

Beans and rice are the base of the most universal legume-grain combination. Here's my own favorite recipe.

Not Just Rice
rice
beans (select your own favorite)
tomato, fresh and cut into small cubes
tree ears (mushroom-like fungus
    that grows on trees)
olive oil
tamari

The rice is the major ingredient; beans, tomato, and tree ears are lesser ingredients. But the exact amount of each is up to you. Cook the rice and beans separately.

The tree ears are packaged in dried form and need to be soaked in hot water for ten minutes. Combine the cooked rice, beans, and tree ears with the tomato. Dress sparingly with olive oil and tamari so there is not a pool of liquid on the bottom of the plate.

Legumes are important enough to be in their own category in the Family of Foods. They are important, but in moderate amounts. Enjoy them in their full variety, and do not overdo any one.

Dairy Products

The human body needs at least 800 to 1,200 mg of calcium per day for its mechanical and chemical infrastructure. It helps to include a dairy product in your diet each day to assure adequate calcium intake. To hold down the saturated fat and the calorie count, use the nonfat variety. In most recipes requiring milk, nonfat milk works well. Yogurt, or yogurt thickened by draining some of the whey, can often substitute for sour cream. Yogurt alone is a good snack and makes a significant contribution to a meal. If the taste of plain yogurt is too tart for you, add one teaspoonful of maple syrup. The maple syrup remains quite fluid even when cold, and mixes easily to flavor the whole cup of yogurt. Chopped up fresh fruit (apple, pear, melon, or berries) is another alternative, and you can be more generous with the fruit than with the maple syrup. Yogurt, with a calcium content of over 400 mg (per eight ounces of the plain, low-fat variety) plus active cultures of Lactobacillus, is a special, almost magical food.

Hard cheeses inherently have a high fat content. Yet, they offer distinctive flavors that have no low-fat equivalent. The solution to the quandary is to use highly flavored cheeses in grated form. A small amount of grated cheese goes a long way for taste. A level tablespoonful of coarsely grated Romano weighs about one-half ounce, which does not add up to much fat or many calories. Romano or Parmesan adds taste to various casseroles, rice recipes, and pasta dishes. The grated cheese also contributes a little protein and a little calcium.

Animal Proteins

Meat and Poultry. The way to keep animal protein foods sparse in your diet is to consider them as a minor ingredient in entree recipes. If the animal protein is prepared as a separate dish, the portion should be small enough to serve as a complement to the main course. A modest amount of meat or fowl, added to an entree whose main ingredients are grains and vegetables, gives that dish added character and taste. The meat in such amounts does not add substantial fat or calories.

Eggs. Eggs are a key ingredient in many recipes that can add variety to your diet. Compare the number of eggs in the recipe to the number of servings the recipe yields, and stay within the guidelines of two or three eggs a week, one at a sitting.

Seafood. Fish and shellfish, if caught in relatively unpolluted waters, can be eaten in greater amounts than meat and poultry. If using canned fish, such as tuna and salmon, be sure it is packed in water rather than in oil.

Fresh or frozen fish can be prepared in different ways: baking, broiling, poaching, stewing, and frying (not deep frying). If the fish is very fresh, a little lemon juice and ground pepper is all the help it needs. Broiled fish is best prepared in this way.

For whole flat fish—such as flounder and sole—and for filets of any other fish that is very mild, I use a semipoaching technique in a cast iron pan. Lightly coat the well-seasoned cast iron pan with a teaspoon of canola oil and heat with a medium flame. Place the fish in the pan and move it side to side for the first minute to prevent sticking. Then add dry white wine to cover the bottom of the pan and allow to simmer. While the bottom of the fish is cooking, baste the top a bit and add ground pepper or any herbs to your liking. When the first side is done, six to eight minutes depending on the thickness of the fish, use two plastic spatulas to turn the fish over. (With a single spatula it is impossible to turn the fish without splashing. Stainless steel spatulas, especially if they have squared corners, can scratch the cast iron.) Add wine as needed for the second side. Cook for another three to four minutes until done. Serve with lemon or lime. The fish can share equal billing on the menu with vegetables and/or rice.

Shellfish respond well to stir frying in a wok. Here's a basic recipe for squid. It can be adapted easily for other shellfish.

Ginger Squid
2 tsp. canola oil
$\frac{1}{2}$ to 1 tsp. freshly grated ginger
$\frac{1}{3}$ lb. squid, cleaned and cut into bite-sized pieces
$\frac{1}{2}$ tsp. sesame oil
$\frac{1}{2}$ tsp. tamari or shoyu sauce
rice (cooked)
   Yield: 1 serving

Place canola oil and ginger in a wok and simmer at lowest heat for three minutes. Increase heat to moderate, add squid, and stir fry eight to ten minutes until squid is close to done. The liquid will increase during cooking as the squid give up some of their own liquid. Add sesame oil and tamari sauce, and stir fry for two more minutes. (Small squid need relatively less cooking time.) Remove squid and place on a bed of rice. Reduce liquid and pour over squid and rice. Other vegetables can be added during stir frying. My favorites are water chestnuts and bamboo shoots.

Snacks

Snacks are an important element in the *Aerobic Diet for Reducing*. Snacks can complement a diet or they can undo a diet.

Your need for snacks is determined to a good extent by your lifestyle, especially your meals. Do you skip breakfast? Are the carbohydrates of your meals complex carbohydrates or simple sugars? When do you do your aerobic workouts? How long and strong are they? Whatever your snack needs may be, you must distinguish between beneficial snacks and dangerous ones.

Snacks to Avoid. Snacks that are high in fat and snacks that are high in sugar do not contribute to health but do add to the waistline. Anything deep fried is heavy with fat. Anything breaded and fried in butter, oil, or shortening is heavy in fat. Anything that tastes too sweet surely is. Here's the "be wary" list:

— Potato chips, corn chips, and the like are super-heavyweights. It is easy to rationalize that "a whole bagful weighs only a few ounces." The fat content of an eight-ounce bag of chips can be as much as 12 teaspoons of oil.
— Fries, though not as bad as chips, are still deep fried.
— Croissants and pastries are high in fat. A quick survey of pastry recipes reveals that oil and butter are measured in ½ cups (or greater) more often than in tablespoons. Commonly, a recipe that makes 16 pieces uses ¾ cup of butter.
— A cup of soup makes a nice snack on a winter day. But beware of "cream of" soups which are all high in fat, often three to four times as high as their broth-based counterparts.

- Cheese and crackers sounds healthful. Whole grain crackers supply complex carbohydrates and B vitamins; cheese is rich in protein, calcium, and other nutrients. The problem is that cheese is also high in fat. Cheddar, for example, is 70 percent fat, and others are worse. Cheese and crackers should not be a total snack. Your limit should be two or three small crackers with a minimum of cheese.

- Pizza is another snack that sounds healthy—pizza dough (complex carbohydrate), tomato, and cheese. But the oil and cheese add up to too much fat. Add sausage and pepperoni, and you can forget about any calorie limits at all.

- Ice cream as a snack is doubly ill-advised. It is high in fat and high in sugar. Ice cream contains between 150 and 300 fat calories per cup.

- The so-called "quick energy" candy bars, especially the chocolaty ones, are high in both sugar and fat. Plain chocolate bars, for example, are over 50 percent fat.

- Martinis, no matter how dry, are not a healthful snack. Even an olive at the bottom is not enough of a nutritional saving grace.

The Welcome Snacks. If eight choice snacks are on the minus list, what is left to nourish body and soul at 11 AM and 3 PM? A little thought and imagination generates a list of snacks that will keep you from automatically thinking about doughnuts or Danish pastry. Here's the recommended list:

+ Pretzels are simple and easy. Those made with whole grain flour, or at least part whole grain flour, are the best choice. They are high in complex carbohydrates and low in fat. They are healthier than chips, and crunchier, besides. A four-ounce wineglass of miniature pretzels accompanied by an eight-ounce glass of club soda makes an urbane snack.

+ Peanuts and nuts, if dry roasted, are healthful. Yes, they are by their very nature high in fat, but that fat is mostly unsaturated and thus beneficial. Nuts are easy to overdo, and you need to find a strategy to limit the total. I have found the best way is to use only peanuts and nuts in the shells as a snack. The time and effort in getting them out of the shells automatically limits the numbers.

+ Popcorn is a great snack, and, if you use an herb powder, garlic, or paprika, you will not get the saturated fatty acids or the greasy fingers that come with butter.

+ Fruit is a fine snack. You can bite into apples, pears, and peaches just as they come from the tree, or you can slice the fruit and eat it in style from a porcelain plate. Go first class.

+ Low-fat yogurt is both nutritious and handy as a snack. Diced fresh fruit adds flavor with a minimum of calories.

+ Whole grain flatbreads and crackers are crunchy, low in fat, and low in calories. They come from Scandinavia, Holland, Germany, Ireland, and also the United States. Eat them plain or spread lightly with fruit puree. Another good spread is yogurt cheese, made by draining low-fat yogurt overnight in a cheesecloth-lined colander or sieve.

+ Finger-food veggies are great because they are an all-you-can-eat snack. Try a variety: green beans, celery, fennel, carrots, snow peas, zucchini, and red and green pepper for starters. For a little more zing, make a dip of low-fat yogurt with basil, tarragon, rosemary, thyme, and oregano. Another tasty dip is a red-vegetable puree made from tomatoes and red bell peppers with additions of onion and chopped garlic, all combined together in a blender and seasoned with salt, hot pepper, and cumin seed.

+ Boiled small red potatoes served cold with a pinch of finely chopped parsley and a squeeze of a fresh lemon make a satisfying snack.

+ Ice milk is a healthful substitute for ice cream. So are frozen fruit juice pops that you can make yourself in plastic forms manufactured for the purpose.

You can probably devise many other snacks. Just keep the fat content and the added sugar to a bare minimum.

Trade-Ins

A cook who intends to produce healthful meals must be able to replace a good part of the sugar, fat, and egg yolk content of recipes and menus. Here are a few hints.

o Fruit juice concentrate—apple is preferred—can eliminate much of the sugar in any recipe.

o Broth or dry white wine can replace most of the oil used in stir frying and pan frying.

o Applesauce or prune puree can substitute for some of the oil, butter, and/or margarine in muffin and quick-bread recipes.

o Two egg whites take the place of one of two whole eggs in any recipe. Eggs are included in many recipes for their ability to emulsify or bind ingredients together. Other foods that have this same talent include tapioca, cornstarch, and bananas.

o Fat-free yogurt with added herbs can replace oil-based salad dressings.

o The complete protein of meat can be replaced by plant-based foods with a bit of ingenuity. A vegetable or grain that is missing one of the essential amino acids must be combined with a food that contains that missing nutrient. As a rule of thumb, a grain and a legume usually provide a complete protein. Another strategy is to combine an incomplete vegetable protein with a small amount of an animal-based food. The complete animal protein shares one or more of its essential amino acids with the vegetable protein, yielding a larger amount of complete protein than the two foods taken separately. Here are a few combinations to use:

  o Rice and beans   o Cereal and milk
  o String beans and almonds   o Pasta and clam sauce
  o Bulgur pilaf with tofu   o Buttermilk pancakes

Experiment with these trade-ins and others that you invent yourself. Have fun with low-fat, low-calorie health.

A final trade-in is to develop a liking for a less sweet taste and use less of the sweetening ingredient in the recipe. To give you an idea how easily taste can shift, my friend Abby tells everyone how she changed from two full teaspoons of sugar in her tea to none at all. One day she made a cup of orange spice tea and, while waiting for it to steep, got involved in a telephone conversation. Forgetting that she hadn't added sugar, she took a sip of the tea. She immediately knew that it had no sugar, but she also realized that for the first time she was tasting the true flavor of the tea. Besides, she was saving almost 40 calories. Win, win!

The *Aerobic Diet for Reducing* is a healthful, varied diet. It is not overly restricted, and it requires only that you use fair-sized portions and keep fats and simple sugars to a minimum. Your regular schedule of aerobic walking will keep your metabolism active so that you need not have food and deprivation in the forefront of your thoughts. You will be able to enjoy food, and eating will take its proper place among the activities in your life.

CHAPTER 7

The Aerobic Diet Guide for Maintenance
More Variety, Less Vigilance

Once you have lost enough size and weight, maintenance of your new body does not require a great change in lifestyle. The *Aerobic Diet for Reducing* is the base for the *Aerobic Diet for Maintenance*—except now you can add further variety with additional foods and recipes. You can also increase your caloric intake a little, and there will even be a place for an occasional special treat. What makes it all possible is your regular schedule of aerobic walking—45 minutes, three to four times a week.

You can now expand the Family of Foods to include a few that are somewhat higher in fat content and/or calories:

o Add avocado to the salad veggie list, but be sparing in its use. Avocado is rich in oils and calories and should be used as a complement to the salad rather than as the main ingredient.
o Add olives to the salad list in the same sparing way—no more than four in a serving.
o Add nuts and seeds to the grains list. Measure them out by the teaspoonful.
o Add chick peas to the legumes list, to be used in modest amounts.
o Add peanuts to the legumes list, measurable by the teaspoonful as with nuts.

These few additions to your choices of raw materials can enhance many recipes and create others that you would not have considered while you were reducing. Let's scout through the Family of Foods for new possibilities.

Salads

A sprinkling of sunflower seeds, one teaspoon per serving, adds texture and flavor to leafy green salads. Avocado cut into cubes, one or two ounces per serving, adds color and flavor. Four black olives, halved, add visual and taste distinction. My personal preference is not to use avocado and olives together because their flavors are not complementary. Also, your calorie count will be lower if you use only one of these ingredients in a salad.

Constraints on the oil content of salad dressings can be relaxed a little. Here's a standard dressing with herb variations:

Herb Dressing

½ cup olive oil

¼ cup wine vinegar

(or split the ¼ cupful between wine vinegar and freshly squeezed lemon juice)

1 tsp. prepared mustard

3 or 4 pinches dried basil

(rubbed between forefinger and thumb as you sprinkle)

Fresh basil, chopped finely, should replace the dried if possible. Other options are rosemary, thyme, and marjoram.

Mix vigorously with a fork or whisk. One tablespoonful dresses each portion of the salad well. Three teaspoons are the same as one tablespoon, but psychologically may seem like more.

Green and Yellow Vegetables

The toppings for these veggies, such as slivered almonds on green beans or grated cheese on cauliflower, can be used a little more freely. Keep in mind that the dish is green beans with almonds, not vice-versa. Swiss chard can be served with a couple of extra squares of flatbread. The marinade for antipasto vegetables can have a base of olive oil and vinegar instead of the fat-free marinade offered in the *Diet for Reducing*.

Grains

Many recipes for bread, rolls, and pancakes have ingredients and amounts that add up to too many calories for the *Aerobic Diet for Reducing*. Some of the recipes, if not too heavy with fat (or oil), can be used occasionally for the *Aerobic Diet for Maintenance*. Try my favorite pancake recipe for a weekend brunch.

Apple Yogurt Pancakes

1 cup whole wheat flour
½ tsp. baking soda
2 pinches salt
1 egg
½ cup low-fat yogurt
½ cup low-fat milk
1 tbs. maple syrup
1 tbs. melted butter
1 tbs. mashed ripe banana
1 apple, peeled, cored, thinly
    sliced and cut into 1-inch squares
5 drops vegetable oil (canola oil preferred)

Mix dry ingredients. Mix wet ingredients. Thoroughly mix dry into wet. Wipe cast iron frying pans (I use two at a time) with the vegetable oil. Spoon batter, two tablespoons per pancake, onto hot pans. When bubbles appear on surface, turn pancakes over. Serve with honey, maple syrup, or fruit puree. Yield: 15 pancakes, 3½ inches in diameter.

Seeds and nuts, which are like grains in their amino acid composition, have been added to the grains category for the *Aerobic Diet for Maintenance*. Nuts and seeds are high in protein, but also high in fat and calories. When used with vegetable or fruit dishes, use them sparingly—two teaspoonsful of nuts or a teaspoonful of seeds per serving.

Fruits

Fruit salad with yogurt dressing can be made more interesting with two teaspoonsful of chopped nuts. Whole or chopped raisins can also be added in the same quantity. A large fruit salad should be counted as two servings of fruit.

The three daily servings of fruit recommended for the *Aerobic Diet for Reducing* can now be increased to four in your *Maintenance Diet*. Fruit makes a good snack. If you are going to do a strong workout, a fresh orange an hour before seems to help endurance.

Starchy Vegetables

Starchy vegetables have traditionally been served with butter. In the *Aerobic Diet for Maintenance,* butter is not a four-letter word. A pat of butter on parsleyed potatoes or on a baked potato adds a flavor that is hard to match. Note that a *pat* is no thicker than a quarter inch. A half-inch thick portion of butter is called a *slab*.

Legumes

Chick peas are highly caloric and were not included in the *Aerobic Diet for Reducing*. For your *Maintenance Diet* you can occasionally use modest amounts of them. One way is simply to scatter a few (one tablespoon maximum) on a salad. Chick peas can also be used in the form of hummus, a tasty pâté spread that goes well on pita bread. Hummus contains, besides chick peas, tahini sesame, which has a high oil content. These ingredients place hummus in the occasional treat class.

Peanuts are high in fat content and calories, but they are a good source of protein. Use peanuts in moderation.

Peanut butter made from freshly ground peanuts and nothing else is the best kind for health. The commercial kind is too often hydrogenated, creating a saturated oil. Saturated fats, whether in peanut butter or prime beef, are a health hazard.

Peanut butter can be made into a sauce to use on rice or vegetables. It is especially good on blanched collard greens, a vegetable that traditionally has received help in the taste department from ham or bacon bits. This sauce can also be spread on lean cuts of beef during barbecuing.

Peanut Ginger Sauce
½ cup stock (vegetable- or chicken-based)
2 tbs. peanut butter
1 tsp. grated ginger
½ tsp. tamari

Combine in a saucepan, simmer for 10 minutes, and it's ready to spread. Yield: 8 to 10 servings. Use one tablespoon per serving.

A last note on peanuts is one of caution. Peanuts that have been damaged are vulnerable to attack from a carcinotoxin-producing mold. Less than perfect peanuts are often consigned to the peanut butter plant. It pays to know the integrity of the producer. An alternative is to use almond butter in the same modest quantities.

Dairy Products

Dairy products should be low-fat or nonfat even in a *Maintenance Diet*. The one exception is the use of a small amount of butter for a shellfish recipe or on a cooked vegetable as an occasional taste treat.

Low-fat or fat-free yogurt is again recommended as a source of calcium and complete protein. An occasional extra cup of yogurt per day is no problem in your *Maintenance Diet*.

Animal Proteins

Follow the counsel of the *Aerobic Diet for Reducing* as closely as possible. Meat or poultry still should be a complement to grains and vegetables as an entree, not vice versa.

Limit eggs to three a week, one at any meal.

Seafood twice a week is still advised. Each portion can be up to a third of a pound.

Snacks

The Snacks List in the *Aerobic Diet for Reducing* has enough variety to get you through all the days of the week.

Deep fried anything is still off limits for reasons of health as much as for reasons of weight/size loss.

———————————

Once you have become lean, the transition from the *Diet for Reducing* to the *Diet for Maintenance* is easy and pleasant. The *Diet for Maintenance* is hardly a diet in the usual sense. It is just healthy, enjoyable eating as part of a normal lifestyle.

CHAPTER 8

Health
Illness and Wellness

Many people are interested in losing weight and reducing size for esthetic reasons. Those who are substantially overweight know that reducing is also medically important. They realize, deep down at least, that their current state of being is inimicable to health and long life.

Whether a person is slightly large or very large, effective therapeutic intervention for both health and weight loss requires no drugs and no scalpels. The prescription is, simply, walking.

Health is primary in all our lives. The idioms and expressions of our language, "health and welfare," "health and happiness," and "healthy, wealthy, and wise"—tell us that health always comes first.

The prescription for health was first written by Hippocrates, the Father of Medicine. He said, "If we could give every individual the right amount of nourishment and exercise, not too little and not too much, we will have found the surest way to health."

For most of the twentieth century, health and nutrition have gone hand in hand. The proponents of "you are what you eat" brought their message to the public in the 1920s and 1930s. A number of their hypotheses have recently been validated by scientists who have unlocked a few of the secrets of our bodies' biochemical genius.

Exercise as Medicine

The exercise physiologists, focusing on the second item in Hippocrates' prescription, have found that exercise can have a telling effect on our health. We now know that when a significant amount of muscle is properly used in aerobic exercise, important changes occur in the body's hormones and enzymes and in chemical reactions of many kinds of cells and tissues. If the exercise is sufficient, but not excessive, all of these changes are beneficial.

Let's look into the effects of aerobic exercise, specifically aerobic walking, as it affects the body chemistry of the following medical conditions:

o Hypertension

o Diabetes

o Heart disease

o Respiratory disease

o Arthritis

o Osteoporosis

o Obesity

Hypertension

It is important to have normal blood pressure. High blood pressure not only increases the risk of a stroke, it increases the work of the heart. Over a period of a few years, a heart that must contract with more force to overcome a high diastolic pressure (the pressure between beats) develops thicker walls. The thicker walls are often produced at the expense of the chambers of the heart, especially the left ventricle. Late in the disease, dilation may occur, further limiting the capacity of the muscle to pump blood.

A few investigators, both physicians and exercise physiologists, have studied the effect of exercise on blood pressure. Most of the studies conclude that aerobic exercise lowers blood pressure and that the effect is independent of weight loss. A few studies found exercise to have no effect on mild hypertension. In examining the design of these doubting studies, however, it can be seen that most of them used subjects who were only marginally hypertensive. Some clinicians have suggested that these subjects may well have been normotensive in the first place. We know that aerobic exercise does not affect normal blood pressures. The consensus is that patients with definite hypertensive blood pressures show definite response to exercise. It has also been observed that hypertensive blood pressures start to decline very early in an exercise program, well before changes in resting pulse rate or total cholesterol.

My own experience with hypertensive individuals is that blood pressures come down rapidly once aerobic thresholds of distance, intensity, and frequency are approached. A typical example is Sally, a 56-year-old participant in a walking clinic series that I instructed for a hospital-based weight-loss program in New Jersey. She had hypertension, but her mind was focussed more on the tape measure than on the blood pressure gauge. At the seventh week of the program she went to her physician's office for a regular check-up. He noted how energetic she seemed. He took her blood pressure and was surprised to find that it was normal. Previously it had been unstable and was never satisfactorily controlled with medication. She told him that she was taking a special course in aerobic walking. The doctor said he did not know that there was anything special about walking, but whatever she was doing, she should bottle it. The last I heard, she was working with him to wean herself off the anti-hypertensive medication.

Many other hypertensive individuals have brought their blood pressures down with aerobic walking and, under their physician's guidance, have been able to stop all drug use. It is a good goal. All four classes of antihypertensive drugs can have serious side effects.

Diuretics create mischief with kidney function, and most of the drugs in this class result in potassium loss. Potassium—the very element that would protect against a stroke.

The beta blockers, which are used to control dysrhythmias as well as hypertension, may cause fatigue, sleep disturbances, loss of sex drive, a drop in high density lipoproteins, and reduced cardiac output. The beta blockers are also notorious for reducing maximal exercise performance in terms of duration and speed.

The ACE (angiotensin converting enzyme) inhibitors may produce headaches, dizziness, gastrointestinal distress, low sodium and high potassium blood levels, and bone marrow depression.

The calcium channel blockers may induce nervousness, confusion, headache, insomnia, muscle weakness, urinary tract disturbances, nasal congestion, and more.

The side effects of these drugs are common enough to be a concern. The side effects of walking, in contrast, include the reduction of cardiac risk factors, increase in endurance, and increase in energy levels. Walking is the drug of choice.

Diabetes

Carbohydrate metabolism is critical for diabetics. The blood is the transfer agent for the basic carbohydrate molecule, glucose. In order to maintain a stable blood glucose level, the body must have mechanisms for preventing the blood stream from becoming overloaded or depleted. And it does.

Insulin, produced by the islet cells of the pancreas, is one of the principal mechanisms for preventing the blood from turning into syrup. If the body cannot produce enough insulin, diabetes results and the patient must have supplementary insulin each day. Insulin binds to the cell receptors of different tissues that then utilize the blood glucose in their metabolic processes. In diabetes, either not enough insulin is produced or the insulin receptors are not doing their job.

Insulin-dependent diabetes (IDDM) is called type I. Non-insulin-dependent diabetes (NIDDM) is called type II. Diabetic patients of both types can, by their own efforts, help stabilize their blood sugar levels. They can do something about the supply side of the balance—diet; and they can do something about the utilization side—exercise.

A diet to keep blood sugar on an even line, with no hyperglycemic peaks and no hypoglycemic valleys, is basically the same as the *Diet for Maintenance*. Diabetics just have to keep a closer watch on balancing energy intake with energy output. The *Diet for Maintenance*, you recall, stays away from the simple sugars that would flood the blood with glucose.

Exercise is more complicated in its effect on blood glucose. The following physiologic mechanisms all tend to keep glucose from accumulating too rapidly in the blood of diabetics of both type I and type II, as well as in normal people.

o Exercising muscles use 7 to 20 times more glucose in their energy cycles than at rest.

o Exercise-trained individuals have a greater percentage of lean tissue, which is metabolically more active than fat.

o Exercise-trained individuals can store more glucose in the form of liver and muscle glycogen.

o Exercise-trained individuals have greater numbers of actively working insulin receptors in the tissues of their bodies. These receptors bind insulin, which stimulates the cells to increase the utilization of glucose.

The above changes are true in both type I and type II diabetics, as well as in normal individuals.

Type I. Insulin-dependent diabetics who are aerobically trained can reduce their insulin requirements by 20 percent or more, depending on the level of exercise. Type I diabetics who are physically active have been shown to be less likely to develop macrovascular eye disease in later life. Other studies have shown that diabetics who currently have higher levels of physical activity exhibit fewer cardiovascular complications overall.

Insulin-dependent diabetics must be careful with exercise. Strenuous exercise when blood glucose levels are low can reduce those levels further. Exercising when blood glucose levels are high (over 300 mg per 100 ml of blood) can cause a further rise in blood glucose. Strenuous exercise at a time when insulin activity is high can cause a precipitous fall in blood glucose. A few rules will help:

o Monitor blood sugar both before and after exercise.

o Do not exercise when blood sugar is below 60 mg per 100 ml or above 300 mg per 100 ml.

o Have a snack (complex carbohydrate) an hour or two before exercise.

o Have food (complex carbohydrate) every two or three hours after exercise up until bedtime.

o In consultation with your physician, reduce insulin dosage appropriately, paying attention to the time of day that you exercise and the time of peak insulin activity.

o Do not inject insulin into a muscle that will be used in exercise. Insulin absorption will be accelerated by the increased blood flow to the exercising muscle.

o Learn how your body responds to insulin and exercise, both in degree and in timing. Let your physician know, too.

If you are insulin dependent, you are probably careful with your diet and diligent about taking insulin. The above exercise precautions will be easy for you to follow. As you learn how your body responds, they will become easier yet. Type I diabetes is no bar to exercise. Indeed, many diabetic athletes have performed at professional and world class levels.

Type II. Non-insulin-dependent diabetics also benefit from exercise, and for the same reasons. Studies have shown increased insulin binding in both muscle cells and blood cells of exercising subjects. Other tissues, as well, are likely to have increased insulin receptor activity.

The effect of exercise in type II diabetes is often significant enough to control blood sugar without the use of oral medication or supplemental insulin. In some individuals, exercise exerts such a strong effect that taking antidiabetic agents concomitantly can drop blood sugar levels into a hypoglycemic range.

If exercise can control type II diabetes so well that no drugs are needed, can it prevent the disease altogether? The answer is a resounding, "Yes." In a study of almost 6,000 University of Pennsylvania alumni, Susan P. Helmrich and her co-investigators concluded, "Increased physical activity is effective in preventing NIDDM, and the protective effect is especially pronounced in persons at the highest risk for the disease."

Although type II diabetes is not as unstable as type I and there is less risk of a precipitous fall or steep rise in blood sugar levels, it is still prudent to avoid exercise extremes, especially when first going into an exercise program.

Heart Diseases

Heart disease comes in different forms:

1. Coronary artery disease (narrowing of the arteries that supply blood to the tissues of the heart)
2. Valvular disease (pathological changes in the valves which normally permit the blood to flow freely, and in the proper direction, through the four chambers of the heart)
3. Dysrhythmias (electrical disturbances resulting in heartbeat irregularities)
4. Cardiomyopathy (weakness of the cardiac muscle)

These forms of heart disease are not mutually independent. Each can influence one or two of the others, and the influence is not for the better. Other conditions such as thyroid disease, hypertension, and faulty lipid metabolism may also influence heart function adversely.

These are only the basics. The complete details are enough to make a cardiologist look to heaven in a plea for insight.

Coronary Artery Disease. Many studies have been done to define the relationship between exercise and heart disease, most of them concerned with coronary heart disease. Most of the large cross-sectional studies have shown a lower risk of heart attack in individuals who are physically active. Other studies have compared heart attack survivors whose rehabilitation included endurance exercise with the survivors who remained inactive in their daily life.

Roy J. Shephard at the University of Toronto reviewed nine major studies done around the world. In seven of the nine studies, patients who had undergone programs of progressive endurance exercise had a 20 percent to 50 percent better survival rate than those who received only medical care. The pooled data showed that the mortality rate was reduced by an average of close to 30 percent.

Animal studies have noted parallel findings in the development of coronary heart disease (Kramsch). A 42-month study of monkeys examined the effect of diet and exercise on the size of the coronary arteries. The sedentary animals on a high-fat and high-cholesterol diet had arteries that were the most constricted. The sedentary animals on a normal diet had average-sized arteries. The exercised animals on a high-fat and high-cholesterol diet had arteries that were the most open. We can only hypothesize about the status of the coronary arteries in exercised animals on a normal diet.

Other animal studies have shown that exercise training increases coronary artery blood flow and also increases the number of capillaries that supply the heart muscle.

Studies in both animals and humans have found that exercise improves lipid metabolism, resulting in:

o Lower levels of total cholesterol

o Lower levels of serum triglycerides

o Lower levels of low density lipoproteins

o Higher levels of high density lipoproteins

All of these improvements contribute to a lower risk of coronary artery blockage. Overall we must conclude that aerobic levels of exercise help to keep our coronary arteries healthy.

Valvular Disease. When it comes to valvular heart disease, the rules are changed. Faulty valves may be the result of a long-ago bout of infection, a congenital deformity, or something else that can not be traced. Exercise will not bring normal anatomy to the leaflets of a distorted valve. Indeed, valve dysfunction can limit exercise performance.

Dysrhythmias. Little research has been done to determine the effect of exercise on dysrhythmias. Theoretically though, aerobic exercise should help. We know that adrenalin can set off a sensitized heart and that endurance exercise reduces and stabilizes catecholamine (adrenalin and noradrenalin) levels. Logic suggests that exercise might well reduce the likelihood of dysrhythmias and, if they did occur, lessen their severity.

As with other types of heart disease, you need your physician's guidance. He or she needs to know that your walking program is a graduated one, building up to aerobic levels over a period of several weeks. You must remember to do a proper warmup before every workout, especially avoiding cold starts at full pace.

Cardiomyopathy. Cardiomyopathy is a disease of the heart muscle fibers, often resulting in heart failure. In cardiomyopathy, the cardiac muscle cells do not respond normally to stress or exercise challenge. An exercise program should be modest to moderate, and the gradual increases in distance and intensity should be *very* gradual. Walking is the ideal exercise for such individuals. Consult with your physician to determine the distance at which to start and the incremental increases in distance and pace over the subsequent weeks.

Respiratory Disease

With exercise, the increased oxygen demands are met by:

1. Increased pulmonary function
2. Increased cardiac output
3. Increased blood flow to the muscles

The lungs can, on demand, increase air exchange by 15 times. That is more than enough to fully oxygenate the blood that the right side of the heart is pumping through the lung field. The heart can increase its output by a maximum of only seven times when it is called on to deliver more blood to exercising muscles.

Chronic Obstructive Pulmonary Disease (COPD). Pulmonary function in COPD is markedly restricted. A pair of lungs so afflicted may be able to deliver less than a four-fold increase in oxygen upon exercise. Neither can such lungs adequately discard the carbon dioxide formed in the exercise energy cycles. The breathlessness from the combination of carbon dioxide accumulation and oxygen deficit severely limits exercise performance.

Yet, exercise will improve fitness levels. As the walking program progresses the COPD sufferer is able to walk further and faster and experiences less respiratory distress. The improvement carries over to the physical tasks of daily life. Aerobic walking at moderate levels is the ideal exercise. It is important to increase distance and speed very gradually over a period of several weeks and to be patient with the rate of improvement. If you have COPD, your physician should advise you on starting distance and rate of progress.

Asthma. Asthma involves disparate components—inflammation or infection, allergy to environmental agents, and stress and anxiety. It is episodic, appearing when all the precipitating factors gang up to constrict the oxygen supply.

It is well known that strenuous exercise can bring on a bout of asthma, but no serious study has been made of the beneficial effect of exercise on asthma.

I can report the experience of four individuals, each with a well-documented history of asthma, who have had instruction in aerobic walking. Three of the four began walking for general fitness and weight loss, but coincidentally noted a marked improvement in their asthma status. The fourth started walking specifically for his asthmatic condition at my suggestion and is now able to engage in more strenuous daily activities without precipitating an attack. All four now use much less medication and feel less at risk. Although the physiological mechanisms for this improvement are not entirely clear, we know that exercise affects the body's adrenalin and cortisone chemistry and influences its immune response, all of which affect pulmonary function. Can aerobic walking be a new and effective treatment for asthma? The research needs to be done.

Arthritis

Arthritis victims often consider themselves just that—victims. They feel powerless against their disease and allow their pain and limited range of motion to restrict all physical activity.

The two most prevalent forms—osteoarthritis and rheumatoid arthritis—are separate diseases. Rheumatoid arthritis is an affliction of connective tissue metabolism and includes an inflammatory component. Osteoarthritis is a disease of aging and of wear and tear on the joints.

Despite the differences, both types of arthritis can benefit from exercise. Studies have shown that arthritic patients can exercise and do improve their levels of aerobic fitness, walking speed, and daily physical activity. Investigators in Scandinavia have reported that rheumatoid arthritis subjects were able to achieve true aerobic levels of exercise without distress to their joints (Minor).

The Malkin Technique of aerobic walking is more fluid than ordinary brisk walking and places less pressure on the joints of the body. Arthritic stiffness and limited range of motion not prevent learning the technique or making gains in fitness. It's worth a nice, easy try.

Osteoporosis

Dietary calcium can remineralize osteoporotic bones, but only if exercise stimulates the bones to incorporate the mineral into their structure. It also helps to have optimal levels of other minerals, nutrients, and hormones.

The calcium content of the blood serum is even more important to the normal functioning of the body than the calcium of the bones. The calcium of the blood and body fluids is responsible for blood clotting, nerve and muscle function, and other high level activities. The body's priority is to guard the blood level of calcium. If there is not enough supplied from the diet, the body takes it from the bones.

Calcium metabolism is highly complex and is influenced by many factors: dietary calcium, calcium absorption, calcium excretion, vitamin D, estrogen and testosterone, parathyroid hormone, cortisone, growth hormone, prostaglandins, calcitonin, phosphorus, magnesium, fluoride, alcohol consumption, and exercise. These factors are not mutually exclusive. Rather, each may work with or against one or more of the others.

The most important factors for women are dietary calcium, estrogen, and exercise.

The calcium requirement for premenopausal women is about 1,000 mg per day. Estrogen-deficient women need about 1,500 mg per day. Some diet surveys report that the average diet of middle-aged American women supplies only about 500 mg per day. Supplements are often advisable.

Estrogen in women is necessary not only for reproductive function, but also for calcium metabolism. When estrogen levels decline, as in menopause, bone resorption increases. After a few years the bone loss may be significant enough to incur the risk of a fracture.

Estrogen replacement, in many cases, is a logical solution to the problems of menopause. It not only helps to stop the bone mineral decline, it also addresses the other unpleasant symptoms of menopause. Hormone replacement therapy must be monitored carefully, and a physician's attention is needed.

Exercise, when dietary calcium and estrogen levels are adequate, will increase bone density significantly. Endurance and resistance exercises are both effective. The opposite effect—demineralization of bone—is seen with enforced bed rest and conditions of weightlessness.

Those not yet menopausal have a chance to build stronger bones now. When menopause does arrive, they will be starting with more calcium in the bone bank. Continuing to exercise through and after menopause can slow down the resorption process considerably. Many investigators have studied the bone-mineral response to exercise in relationship with the other influences on calcium metabolism. Exercise consistently helped either to increase bone density or slow down the rate of reabsorption.

Calcium, exercise, and estrogen all are important. Although a physician is needed when it comes to estrogen replacement, a woman can be her own physician as far as exercise and nutrition are concerned. The prescriptions to write are:

o Maintain adequate calcium intake by means of diet and, if need be, supplements.

o Maintain a regular schedule of workouts (three to four times a week) at a fairly strong pace. In each workout, the number of rhythmic, repetitive strides and the magnitude of force behind each stride both stimulate bone; but magnitude counts more. A strong workout for 45 minutes is much better than a longer workout at an easy, comfortable pace.

Whether pre- or postmenopausal, a woman does not have to yield to osteoporosis.

Obesity

Obesity is considered a metabolic disorder, but the medical profession has not been very successful in treating this condition. It is tough to fight against heredity, metabolism, and a hearty appetite.

The size of an individual may be extreme, but the problem came about by way of small daily or weekly additions of fat over an *extended* period of time. The proper solution should be in kind— every day, every week over an extended period of time. Aerobic walking three or four times a week, can do what drugs cannot do— it can be used long term, and all its side effects are positive.

o Aerobic walking changes both metabolism and level of activity and lowers the body's set point for weight.

o Aerobic walking is easy on the musculoskeletal system, even for a heavyweight.

o Aerobic walking allows you to enjoy a diet that is not harshly restrictive while losing size and weight.

o After you have reached your goal weight or size, aerobic walking makes the transition to a regular diet so smooth that there is no tendency to go back to binge and starve cycles, or worse.

o Aerobic walking provides a maintenance metabolism that keeps you in good shape esthetically and medically, and allows you three meals a day on a healthful diet.

o Aerobic walking keeps your appetite in line with the caloric requirements of a thinner body.

o Aerobic walking grants emotional stability, raises self-esteem, and helps prevent both depression and anxiety.

o Aerobic walking bestows higher energy levels and increases walking speed. You will move like a thin person, not only in your workouts but also in daily activities.

o Aerobic walking changes self-image to that of a slimmer person. Those who lose weight by means of extreme diets still think of themselves as fat. Only by having the metabolism of a thinner person is there a thinner self-image.

Exercise for Wellness

Treatment of medical conditions constitutes only half of health care—the illness half. The other half is wellness, or the resistance to disease. Exercise can strengthen your immune system to fight off the physical, chemical, bacterial, and viral enemies that we come in contact with every day. Exercise creates a highly efficient circulatory system in which the heart easily supplies blood to all the vital organs. Exercise creates a better balance between the sympathetic (fight or flight) and parasympathetic (rest and repair) nervous systems so that your body responds in the most healthful way to different situations and stresses. Exercise promotes efficiency throughout the system of endocrine glands of the body. In short, your body becomes resistant to illness. Further, you *feel* healthier and more vibrant.

Aerobic walking brings together both halves of the health apple, and adds a little spice in doing so. Aerobic walking is the future of health care, and it does not have to wait for the future.

CHAPTER 9

Perqs
Beyond Health and Weight Loss

Most people exercise for reasons of health or slimness, but there are many other benefits that come along with no additional effort. Let us call them perquisites. You even may find one of them to be as important as your original reasons.

Places to Go, Things to See

Aerobic walk training has special advantages when visiting places away from home. You will have higher energy levels and not become weary from a day's exploring, whether the exploring is in a National Park or the galleries of a museum.

Walking from place to place in a city provides a chance to see small details, and there is time for images to sink into your memory bank. In a car, there are only fleeting glances. In rural areas walkers can go many places where cars cannot.

On a visit to Paris some years ago, I stayed at a small hotel on the Île de la Cité, an island in the middle of the River Seine, and walked everywhere in the city. One day when the sky was covered with impressionist-painted clouds, I walked along the Seine and around to that marvel of French engineering, the Tour Eiffel. I spent an hour looking at the great iron structure from different sides and taking a few photos from the best angles. A bus pulled up, bringing 25 or 30 tourists who were visiting the city's attractions. As they left the bus, the tour leader instructed his charges, "You have only five minutes, so take your pictures and get back to the bus quickly. We're a bit behind schedule."

The Eiffel Tower was one of the few sights the tour group stopped to see. Most of the City of Lights had to be seen through the bus windows. In contrast, I spent as much time as I wanted at the Eiffel Tower. On the way back, I browsed in book stalls, watched an old man fishing in the Seine, and stopped to say *"Bonjour"* to a merchant tending her cart in the flower district.

In Paris, fitness has advantages both outdoors and indoors. The Louvre Museum has miles of gallery space, and spending four or five hours on one's feet enjoying centuries of art requires stamina that only aerobic walking can provide.

Other cities have their own features that are best discovered on foot. Amsterdam is a city that I explored almost entirely by leg power. It is a city that seems to have been designed for walking. The streets along the canals are delightful, their buildings often dating back to before our Revolutionary War. Walking along the canals, I came across a Delftware shop with centuries-old blue tiles in the window. Then, the Riiksmuseum, with its collection of Rembrandt's paintings invited further hours of walking.

I also recommend Florence, Rome, London, New York, and Washington at a pedestrian's pace. With strong legs and lungs you will get a more intimate view of each city.

In the countryside, walking skills can be even more vital. Walking trails are everywhere. Some of them, such as the Appalachian Trail and the Pacific Crest Trail, are in the National Great Trails system. Every state has many trails that may be less well known but just as scenic. They range from flat shore trails to steep mountain trails,

In Boulder, Colorado, it is possible to walk from the western edge of town right into the Rockies. During one of the International Pedestrian Conferences held annually in Boulder, I signed on for a hike to Royal Arch, a natural rock arch high above the city. The Arch can be seen from the trail only when you are almost upon it, and so if you turn back early, you do not get to see it at all. It is less than a day's trek there and back, but, with rough terrain in places, it is a fair challenge. At a point about two hours out, eight of the original fifteen hikers decided to head back. They felt that four hours was their limit for the day's excursion. We hardy ones pushed on and made it to the Royal Arch. The sight of it overlooking the plains to the east was ample reward. On our return, at an easier pace, we seemed to walk more lightly.

In the Northeast, the valley of the Upper Delaware River is a special place to visit. It is special for canoeists, and it is special for walkers. The Upper Delaware begins at Hancock, New York, and retains its character for 75 miles to Port Jervis where the three states—New York, New Jersey, and Pennsylvania—meet. The Upper Delaware is almost a secret, compared to the well-known Delaware Water Gap further south. The Upper River is narrow enough to feel like a personal river. There are rapids in many places and occasional eddies at others. The banks are generally steep, but in many places it is possible to walk to the water's edge. Water birds are common, and, with luck, you may see a bald eagle overhead. Several trails along the Upper Delaware not only provide wonderful views but allow visitors to feel a part of this special river.

Five miles south of Narrowsburg, a trail runs alongside the Ten Mile River tributary to where it enters the Delaware. Then the trail crosses a stone arch bridge to follow the Delaware north to the railroad trestle. It is an easy two or three hour jaunt out and back.

On another day, cross the Narrowsburg Bridge to the Pennsylvania side and walk north on River Road to to Skinner's Falls at Milanville. River Road is a little-used blacktop road with many curves and many ups and downs. For most of its seven miles, you can look down to the moving River. At Skinner's Falls you can cross the Milanville Bridge to the New York side and cool your feet in the River.

If you are in good shape, these Upper Delaware River walks are doubly pleasant—scenic and exhilarating

In the Caribbean, long beaches abound. What can be more dreamy than strolling along aqua-blue waters on a powder sand beach where yours are the only footprints from one end to the other? My favorite Islands are Virgin Gorda, Bequia, Vieques, Anguilla, Nevis, and Granada, and all have great walking beaches.

The island of Montserrat has few beaches. Rather, it is volcanic with lush rain forests. A spectacular destination is La Souffriere, the boiling sulfur springs, high in the mountains. The trek begins as a pleasant walk in the shade of tropical trees and ends at a treeless landscape with bubbling hot springs that have randomly broken through the surface and deposited cascades of sulfur crystals. I will remember it for a lifetime.

There are great walks and hikes all over the world, as well as at home in the States. Here is a further sampling that I can personally recommend:

o Baxter State Park and Mount Katahdin (Maine)
o Cadillac Mountain at Acadia National Park (Maine)
o Borestone Mountain (Monson, Maine)
o Squaw Mountain at Moosehead Lake, from the top of the chair lift to the Fire Tower (Maine)
o The Long Trail various sections (Vermont)
o Mad River Glen and Sugarbush (Vermont)
o The Mianus River Gorge (southern Connecticut)
o Watkins Glen (New York)
o Lake Minnewaska in the Shawangunk Mountains (New York)
o The Palisades along the lower Hudson River (New York)
o Fire Island Seashore (New York)
o The Brooklyn Bridge (New York)
o Prospect Park in Brooklyn and Central Park in Manhattan (New York)
o The Great Swamp (New Jersey)
o The Tidal Basin (Washington, D.C.)
o Olympic National Park (Washington)
o Mt. Ranier (Washington)
o The Hoh Rain Forest (Washington)
o The trail to Moon Hole, an impressive natural rock arch (Bequia, West Indies)
o Culebra—the road to the bird sanctuary (Puerto Rico)

And that's just for starters in the Western Hemisphere north of the Equator. You can do a little research yourself. Tourist agencies of every state and region will send you enough information to start your own personal travel agency. The DeLorme Mapping Company (Freeport, Maine 04032) publishes an Atlas and Gazetteer for many states with an emphasis on the outdoors. U. S. Geological survey maps are a wonderful source for finding practically unknown trails and woods roads. With a survey map you can discern streams, waterfalls, ravines, and marshes, and plan a hike accordingly. With legs tuned and stamina high, you will be dauntless.

Neighborhood Safety

In New York, people live with thoughts of personal safety in the front or back of their minds. In sections of Brooklyn far down Flatbush Avenue from Manhattan, they speak of a safe neighborhood. In Brooklyn Heights and Carroll Gardens, they are satisfied to live on a safe street. In Manhattan, they refer to a safe building. A neighborhood, whatever its size, is safer if a "sense of neighborhood" exists, where its residents know who belongs.

In my small neighborhood in Flatbush, I started a walking club to promote health and slimness. An important perq, however, came out of our presence on the streets three times a week, a vigorous presence at that. We became the eyes and ears of the neighborhood.

A group of residents in another "neighborhood," a large apartment building in Manhattan, participated in a series of aerobic walking clinics held in Carl Schurz Park. They became better acquainted as they got together in pairs and small groups for additional workouts between clinic sessions. It added to the cohesiveness of their "neighborhood" and it became known that people of vigor were living there.

A safer neighborhood is only one side of the safety picture. Aerobic walking also improves posture and produces a strong stride. You will be seen as walking with purpose—the very antithesis of a victim. Set an example for others in your neighborhood.

Family Ties

Walking can be a path to family cohesiveness. Hikes and outings for the whole family afford time together. Parents who are highly fit walkers easily keep up with teenagers. In fact, if the kids are not in top shape, such parents are well advised to slow down a bit so their kids will not fall behind. On the trail, members of the family share sights and sounds. There is no need for a constant flow of conversation, and silent stretches are not uncomfortable. Coming upon a rock formation that looks like a giant tortoise or seeing a wild animal is a stimulus to conversation. Share a pleasant experience with someone and you will have pleasant feelings towards that individual. It even applies to children and parents.

If you plan a hike where there are streams to cross or ponds to investigate for tadpoles, it would be wise to pack an extra pair of footwear for children who are curious and adventurous.

Having a destination is always a good idea. Achieving a goal is satisfying and will make selling the next hike easier. If the goal is special, so much the better.

Being walk-trained and fit generates respect from kids, even a bit of pride. My son Devin is in his twenties and athletic, but he does not walk seriously, as I do. Recently he told one of his friends that his father can out-walk and out-run both of them. On a bicycle, however, I'm no match for him. Mutual respect is good.

Family outings need not be limited to you and your children. Three and even four generations can walk together. Smaller kids and older grandparents may be a little slower, but they make a great team. With an extra generation between them, grandparents and grandchildren are often close companions.

Aerobic walking benefits grandparents in all the medical ways discussed in chapter 8. Aerobic walking thus enables a grandparent to be less at medical risk for debilitating injury or illness. Such an individual is more self-sufficient and independent.

Walking also benefits spouses. Sometimes spouses have the same opinion on a particular matter; sometimes their views are divergent. A walk together allows time to talk *and* think. There is no need for an immediate judgment or decision. A workout together is conducive to putting things in perspective. Aerobic walk training also will tone abdominal and back muscles, valuable for the physical side of emotion. Closeness has many facets.

Time Saving

We all move from place to place several times a day. It may be from home to office, to conference room, to private office, to lunch, back to office, and so on. Whatever your occupation, whether in the home or outside, moving from place to place usually involves walking. If you are aerobic walk trained, you will move faster and more easily from one place to another.

I had been taking everyday walking for granted when Linda, one of my former students, reminded me of this perq. I met her recently, six months after she had made aerobic walking part of her lifestyle. She greeted me with news of a great discovery.

"Mort, I'm so glad I took your classes. Aerobic walking has been a savior for me."

I expected to hear about some health benefit she experienced, but she started to talk about algebra. She noted that rate times time equals distance, and distance divided by rate equals time. Time! Of course. Linda's workday typically consisted of several appointments with potential buyers of the products she represented.

"I've gotten so fast at walking that I'm early to my appointments. And if I need to spend an extra few minutes with a client, I can easily make up the time on the way to the next one."

Perhaps it is a health perq after all. Lower stress levels are certainly conducive to higher health levels.

The Secret to Parking
in the City

My mathematician friend, John, taught me the secret of easy parking in Manhattan. Before I became enlightened, I would try to find a parking space within five blocks of my destination, often circling the same few blocks several times. Now I am willing to park up to ten blocks away and walk the extra distance. By doubling the distance, I have increased my chance of finding a space by *four* times. It is magic in accordance with the formula for the area of a circle—area equals pi times radius squared (Πr^2).

It may be simpler to visualize a square, 10 blocks by 10 blocks, with a theatre right in the center. That would be about the size of the area I used to cruise for a parking space—100 square blocks. Now, I search an area of 20 blocks by 20 blocks—ten blocks north, south, east, and west of the same theatre. But 20 by 20 is *400* square blocks—four times the number of potential parking spaces. Walking ten blocks is easy enough for a walker who does three to four mile workouts. It delights me when I find a parking space the first time around, even if it's a larger around. If you, like I, hate circling for a parking space, try Πr^2.

Cross-Training

The strong metabolic effect of aerobic walking is the result of the technique that uses a large total muscle mass as a power source. Working the hamstring, gluteal, and calf muscle groups plus the trunk muscles, add up to a can't-fail exercise.

Most people who do aerobic walking for health and/or weight control find that they also gain a great deal of stamina. It has happened with every one of the thousands of individuals who completed a six- or eight-week course with me. If you enjoy participating in sports that use the large leg and trunk muscles—basketball, football, soccer, boxing, track and field, and others—you will find your performance improved by aerobic walking. The muscles, especially the hamstrings, also gain strength and resiliency and become less vulnerable to injuries.

Two sports, cross-country skiing and snowshoeing, are close to aerobic walking in their biomechanics. Aerobic walk training would be good preparation for an active winter vacation. All too often we go off for a wonderful week in the snow country, ski for a few hours the first day, and can't move our muscles for the rest of the vacation. A couple of strong walking workouts would be preventive medicine.

Conversely, walking can benefit from cross-country skiing. Ray Sharp, after he had set the record for the one-mile walk during a track meet in Madison Square Garden, was asked how he was able to train well enough in the winter months to set a new record at that time of year. He replied that he he had been cross country skiing in the Rockies.

Snowshoeing, too, uses aerobic walking muscles. Snowshoeing is a sport for getting out into the countryside and exploring trailless areas, and the better your endurance the further you can trek. It is one more reason for staying in shape with aerobic walking.

Making Life on the Job Easier

Easing the physical demands of one's occupation may be the most important perquisite of aerobic walking.

Footwork. Many employees would find their jobs easier with legs, lungs, and hearts that were walk trained—police officers, mail carriers, sanitation workers, hotel employees, gardeners, and others who are on their feet for most of the day.

Music Makers. A few years ago I was at the recital of a clarinetist whose program included pieces from the Baroque period, which would show off his technical skills. His fingering was wonderful, but he had to gasp for air between passages. He was clearly overweight and less than fit. In contrast, flutist Eugenia Zuckerman, at a concert series given at the New York Public Library, played difficult pieces with such perfect technique and breath control that she gave the illusion of not needing to breathe while playing extended passages. It turns out that Ms. Zuckerman usually begins her day with an aerobic walking workout. (See the last chapter, "Small Miracles.")

Aerobic walking makes good sense not only for woodwinds but also for brass and vocal performance, all of which need respiratory stamina.

Deals and Deadlines

In the corporate world of conferences and negotiations, stamina counts, especially when deadlines approach. Labor and management negotiators may lock horns in all-night sessions when a contract runs out at midnight and a strike is set for 9 AM. Stamina levels can determine who gives up more and who gives up less in the final agreement.

Deadlines are a monthly event for Dr. Richard Strauss, the editor of the journal, *The Physician and Sportsmedicine*. He does not stay in the editorial offices during lunch hour. Instead, he takes a sandwich and an apple and walks twenty minutes over to a bench under a favorite tree. If the weather is not cooperative, he goes for his walk and has lunch after he returns to the office. He says his lunchtime absence contributes to his secretary's health; she in turn says Dr. Strauss is more mellow and productive in the afternoon following his walk.

Social Forms

Walking and relationships go hand in hand. On a walking date you have ever-changing scenery. You can walk together without conversation, or you can have animated discussion. Silence is not awkward as you share the passing scene. Stopping afterward for iced tea (summer) or hot chocolate (winter), you will still feel the exhilaration of your walk.

Solo workouts in a park filled with other fitness people provide another social pathway. It is easy to make the acquaintance of another walker or, if you are pretty fast, a runner. A smile or a "Hi" feels natural enough.

I sometimes give private lessons to a senior citizen in Alley Pond Park in Queens. Our route is an old carriage road called Vanderbilt Parkway, now reserved for human-powered transport only. Occasionally we see a bright-eyed woman, about my age, who runs the same course. The second time I saw her, we smiled to each other. The third time we both waved. I feel I have a park friend.

In Wilmington, Delaware, a friar named Brother Isidore dresses in a traditional long robe, but wears modern athletic shoes. He makes his rounds throughout the city on foot and, with a kind word, finds friends everywhere. *Walking Magazine* quotes Brother Isidore: "When you're out walking, conversation comes more automatically than it does indoors. People feel freer outdoors." Wisdom from a holy man.

Save the Environment

We all would like to see a cleaner, more healthful environment. Walking can be your environmental issue. Walking for reasonable distances, instead of getting into your car and driving, creates a good deal less pollution. Engineers who work on the problem of air pollution have established that most auto pollution is attributable to short distance stop-and-go driving, especially the first eight minutes after starting your car (the cold-start warmup period). If you need to travel only a mile or so, remember that you are walking much more than that distance in each of your workouts. A mile is no sweat.

You can take a step beyond your own environmental contributions by having others join you in walking for health, weight loss, or any of the other dozen good reasons. Once they are in shape, you can convince them to leave their internal combustion engines home for short distance travel.

If we set a good example for our kids, they will see walking as a way to save the environment. They can spread the idea to their classmates who will go home and badger their parents. You can set off a chain reaction that will culminate in our breathing a little easier.

The Body-Mind Connection

From Aristotle to the British Romantic poets to Albert Einstein, some of civilization's best minds have found that walking is a catalyst for the imagination.

At the school of philosophy he founded in Athens, Aristotle discoursed with his students as they walked together around the covered, outside walls (peripatoi) and into the countryside. The disciples became known as *peripatetics.*

Two millennia later, the British poets of the early nineteenth century knew the effect walking had on stimulating the imagination. Keats described a walk he took with Coleridge: "I walked with him . . . for nearly two miles. In those two miles he broached a thousand things."

Coleridge and Wordsworth were inveterate walkers but had not known each other until Coleridge read Wordsworth's account of his walk across France to the Alps. Coleridge thereupon set off to the Wordsworths' home in Racedown, some forty miles away. William and Dorothy Wordsworth took a liking to their newfound colleague, and the three became good friends. In the years following, they had many walks together, each providing sustenance for the imagination of the other two.

American writers, too, used walking to spark their creative forces. Emerson, Whitman, Thoreau, and many others wrote not only of the human spirit but also of the art of walking. *The Magic of Walking* by Sussman and Goode include several of their essays.

At the turn of the twentieth century, the human imagination turned in force to other formats than literature. Albert Einstein saw the universe, in its smallest and largest dimensions, in novel ways. In working out his elegant new theories, he sometimes found himself at a sticking point. Rather than stare at his equations, he habitually went out for a walk. Afterward, an obvious solution often popped into his head. He soon realized that walking freed him to muse and think in metaphors, the stock-in-trade of the imagination.

For us lesser lights, freeing the imagination is a pleasant perq of walking, even if we don't come up with something as valuable as $E = mc^2$.

In the last half of this century, science began to examine the influence of the body on the mind. Exercise physiologists and psychologists have studied how exercise affects our thought processes and our emotions.

Investigators at the University of Southern California found that aerobic exercise increased the ability of subjects to concentrate and reason logically. At the same time, depression and anxiety were decreased. The control group showed neither of these changes.

A joint study at the University of Texas, the University of Houston, Baylor College of Medicine, and the Veterans Administration Medical Center in Houston monitored three groups of retirement age individuals for a period of four years (Rogers). It was found that the retirees who became physically inactive exhibited reduced cerebral blood flow and scored significantly lower on cognition (thought processing) than their counterparts who were physically active and those of the same age who continued to work.

Intelligence has been divided by the academics into two compartments. Fluid intelligence is a reflection of how the brain cells and pathways transmit their electrical and chemical signals and react to those from other parts of the brain. The theory is that fluid intelligence increases up to adolescence when neural maturation is complete. Thereafter, fluid intelligence is supposed to decline and, indeed, is at lower levels in the older population. Crystallized intelligence receives its input from cultural and educational experiences and theoretically can increase throughout life. The wise men and women among us have always been able to compensate for the decline in fluid intelligence by increasing their crystallized intelligence.

A new perspective on intelligence theory recently has come from three different studies, all showing significantly higher fluid intelligence in physically fit subjects. At Purdue University, crystallized and fluid intelligence were tested in both young and older subjects. Crystallized intelligence was unaffected by exercise. Fluid intelligence improved with exercise, the older group showing the greatest gains! Perhaps it should not have been a surprise. Other studies have shown that mild to moderate depression and anxiety states are relieved by levels of aerobic exercise that produce metabolic change. Indeed, brain chemistry does change with aerobic exercise, and brain chemistry enters into the intelligence equation.

Manna for the Psyche

The changes in brain chemistry that heighten the imagination and quicken thought can also affect attitude and facets of personality. I think you will welcome the changes.

o You will take thousands of steps in a four mile workout and, of necessity, learn patience and tenacity.

o You will understand the certainty of the stepwise completion of what you set out to do, whether it be a pleasurable activity like walking or just plain work.
o You will savor success in achievement rather than competition.
o You will find increased mental energy levels and decreased anxiety.

———————————

Participants in aerobic walking programs have told me of these perqs, and I have seen many of them in my own life. It is an open-ended list to which you can add others that you will surely discover for yourself. There is no end of reasons for making walking part of your lifestyle.

CHAPTER 10

Safely, Safely
Gain Without Pain

Exercise people say, "Exercise will make you healthy." Couch potatoes say, "Exercise leads to injury, and that is unhealthy."

The answer, of course, is to exercise in a manner that is safe enough to avoid injury.

Nicely and *safely* are twins in sports and exercise:

o Nicely, which is made of skill and good form, will lessen the chance of injury.

o Safety basics, such as warmups before and stretches after workouts, keep the musculoskeletal system supple so it can be fine-tuned in technique.

It goes without saying that there is no aerobic benefit if you are injured and sidelined.

Avoiding Injury

Sports and exercise, by their very nature, subject the bones, ligaments, and tendons to incredible forces; challenge the body's metabolic capacity; and ask for a high level of performance from the cardiovascular and respiratory systems. But you can exercise safely, and the ways to do so do not have to lessen the effectiveness of the exercise or the fun.

May the Force Not Be with You

From a musculoskeletal standpoint, aerobic walking is one of the safest of endurance exercises. The smoother the form, the less

161

the force on the bones, muscles, and connective tissues—less than 1.5 times body weight at every footfall.

Running, in contrast, commonly produces forces of 2½ to 5 times body weight at every step. It is an amount of force that the body can withstand only so many times in succession. The figures of 2½ to 5 times body weight represent only the vertical force with which the foot hits the ground. The forces generated *within* tendons and ligaments are considerably higher. The Achilles tendon, for example, develops peak forces of 5.3 to 10 times body weight during running.

Pounding Out the Weekly Miles. A number of studies have correlated the incidence of injuries in runners with their average weekly mileage and found that there is a direct relationship. More miles are related to more injuries. Above 40 miles per week, the injury rate goes into high gear. Also, a *sudden* increase in intensity or distance predisposes a runner to injury.

Kenneth E. Powell and coworkers from National Institutes of Health, Centers for Disease Control, and the Institute for Aerobics Research, reviewing several studies, reported that in any given year injury rates for runners are between 24 percent and 60 percent.

An interesting report by S. E. Robbins and G. J. Gouw of Concordia University in Montreal was at odds with the trend toward more cushioning and more technology in athletic shoes. The authors concluded that runners wearing shoes with protective cushioning and anti-pronation features were injured more frequently than those wearing shoes costing under 40 dollars. The hypothesis was examined in the laboratory, as well. Tests of impact forces that could be tolerated by barefoot subjects versus those wearing running shoes showed that barefoot runners, in order to prevent excessive discomfort on the soles of their feet, adjust their stride so the vertical forces they withstand are less than twice their body weight. Shod subjects felt no discomfort at up to eight times body weight and so had no proprioceptive reason to alter a heavy, pounding running style that can shock the knees and spine even as the feet are protected.

It is notable that in barefoot populations, running injuries are rare. In the United States there is now a higher incidence of running injuries than there was before the advent of high-tech shoes.

Walking, of course, does not generate the abusive forces of running. But the vertical forces in walking can be reduced still further with smooth technique. Fluid technique can lower the force at each footfall from 1.5 times body weight with ordinary brisk walking to 1.1 or 1.2 times body weight with aerobic walking.

Not only does a smooth walking form reduce the likelihood of incurring injury, it helps those who have preexisting knee problems or low back pain. For preventing low back pain or ameliorating existing low back pain, pay special attention to posture and balance.

Little research has been done to assess walking injuries in relation to mileage. It would be prudent, though, to use the guidelines for running safety that advise keeping the weekly mileage of workouts well under 40. Actually, most people can attain and maintain a maximal level of fitness and a minimal level of body fat with less than 20 miles a week.

Single Workout Stress. It is not only weekly mileage that will do you in. A single long, hard workout is enough to harm the musculoskeletal system. A typical marathon, even without a Heartbreak Hill or a Queensboro Bridge causes muscle fiber damage. Several studies of marathoners measured blood levels of creatine kinase before and after the race. Creatine kinase is an enzyme that plays an active role in muscle physiology. When there is damage to muscle cells, CK is released into the serum. Every one of these studies of marathon runners showed striking increases in serum creatine kinase levels, averaging more than *ten times* the pre-race values. Moreover, the high CK levels came down very slowly, with enzyme values still at twice normal values five days after the race.

Direct confirmation of the muscle damage came from muscle tissue studies of marathoners. Calf muscle biopsies taken from runners after a marathon exhibited muscle cell degeneration with accompanying inflammatory changes. The peak of destructive changes occurred one to three days after the race. Not every fiber of the muscle was so affected, but the authors of the study reported that the extent of the pathological changes was extensive, with almost every needle biopsy sample showing some areas of muscle cell deterioration and attendant inflammation.

I can add personal confirmation of the toll that a marathon can take. For two years I was a member of the Marathon Medical Corps for the New York City Marathon. From 2½ hours to 6 hours after the start, a steady parade of hundreds of athletes in distress came to us. One year the weather was cool and there were a number of cases of mild to moderate hypothermia. Blisters, as expected in a long race, were plentiful. But the majority of runners who came through triage had severe muscle spasms—calves, quadriceps, and hamstrings. Stretching and/or massage generally gave relief. I noted a few cases of quadriceps and hamstring spasm in the same individual, which limited our treatment choice to massage. Stretching the quadriceps would have exacerbated the hamstring cramping and vice versa.

Interestingly, walkers—there were 100 to 200 participating each year—never appeared at the medical tents for musculoskeletal problems.

Some investigators looking at the problems of overtraining have suggested that 80 to 90 minutes of a hard workout is probably the upper limit of relative safety for most runners. It is sensible for walkers to use those figures, too.

After a strong workout at any distance, the working muscles are more easily triggered into spasm. During and following exercise, there are large-scale shifts of electrolytes, such as potassium and calcium, between the muscle cell and its surrounding tissue fluids. Potassium ions, for example, move from inside to outside the confines of the cell during exercise and then back into the cell after exercise. There are also significant changes in hydrogen and phosphate ion concentrations as well as in glucose and glycogen levels. Fortunately, we do not have to fine-tune our chemistry. You can prevent cramping by enjoying a diet rich in vegetables, fruits and grains; drinking plenty of liquids before and after workouts; and stretching after workouts. It is important to stretch the muscles that worked the hardest. For walking, the stretches described in chapter 4 will do the trick. Stretch right after your cool-down and again later in the day. And stretch again the next day, even if it is a rest day. When stretching at times other than after a workout, be sure to walk around a little first, just to warm the muscles you are going to stretch.

Unnatural Muscle Contractions

Muscles normally contract and *shorten* as they force our bodies to move in the directions dictated by their origins and insertions on our various bones. These normal muscle dynamics are called *concentric contraction.*

But muscles can also contract and not shorten, as in isometric exercises. Further, muscles can contract and be forced to *lengthen* as in downhill running and walking. This type of contraction is termed *eccentric* and is disfavored by the muscle fibers. Extreme soreness can occur if the eccentric contractions are repeated many times with each contraction resisting a sizable force such as total body weight. A climb uphill involves concentric contraction of the quadriceps and calf muscle groups. The return downhill, where the body is held back at each step, uses eccentric contraction of the quads. Before doing a long climb in the mountains, it is a good idea to do some downhill walking the prior week to prepare your muscles.

Shin Critique

Walkers, though they are fairly safe from musculoskeletal mischief, may experience discomfort from one small set of muscles—the anterior tibial muscles located at the front of the lower leg. About 30 percent of the walkers who are new to aerobic walking are subject to tibial muscle discomfort.

The mechanical action of these muscles is to raise the forefoot. In aerobic walking the muscles do their work at the end of the swing, or recovery, phase in preparation for heel contact with the ground. I have found that, in those walkers who are subject to anterior tibial pain, the muscles begin to act up five or ten minutes after beginning the workout. As the workout is continued, the muscles acclimate and the pain diminishes, especially if the pace is eased a little. The pain is not necessarily an indication of injury; it is just that the muscles are not accustomed to the hard work and are complaining. As progress is made in aerobic walking, the anterior tibial muscles become stronger and more resilient. After several weeks there is no further pain.

I must note the slight possibility that anterior tibial problems can persist. The sports medicine literature contains several reports, mostly by orthopedists, of chronic anterior compartment syndrome with higher than normal pressures within the surrounding muscle sheath.

The first prescription is rest. Then, continued training should be at a lower intensity with more gradual advancement in distance and pace. If the pain does not gradually diminish, a visit to a physician is advised. An orthopedic examination may yield further information to provide guidance in training decisions of how soon and how much.

Blisterless

Muscles, tendons, and bones are relatively strong structures. Skin is thinner. At less than marathon distances, blisters can appear if you do not take proper precautions.

Blisters are generally caused by friction that results in shearing forces within the layers of the skin. Small tears occur that fill with tissue fluid, and there you have a blister.

The movement of the foot within the shoe produces the friction that starts the process. The stronger the horizontal force exerted on the shoe, the more friction is produced.

Here are the ways to outwit friction in aerobic walking:

o Use good technique. The force that you use to propel yourself forward—or propel the earth backward—should be exerted by your heel against the heel counter and the full sole of your foot against the full sole of the shoe. The initial ground contact of the heel should be gentle, and the backward force exerted against the earth should increase gradually as the leg passes under the body's center of gravity. At the end of the stride, do not push off with the ball of the foot and do not grip the ground with your toes. The key is to be as balanced as possible.

o Use a thin layer of Vaseline on the bottom of the toes and on the ball of the foot—just where you expect blisters to be a problem.

o Wear two pairs of thin socks instead of one heavier pair. The inside socks will move across the outside socks rather than across your skin.

You may combine any two or all three of these blister tricks. Or, if your walking technique is smooth and well balanced, that may be enough by itself.

Toenails

Toenail injury is common enough among runners and walkers to deserve some attention. Pressure on the nails from the toebox of the shoe, repeated a few thousand times, can cause capillary bleeding in the nailbed. The nail immediately turns black and blue, and you have a typical case of "black toenail." Unlike a black eye or a bruise elsewhere in the body, black toenails last for months. Better to prevent the injury. Use all of the following tricks and techniques:

o Clip all toenails short. File them on their ends and surfaces so they are neither long nor thickened.

o Use Vaseline on and around the nails. Be generous.

o Wear shoes that are roomy in the toebox in all three dimensions—length, width, and height.

o Use good walking technique and be well balanced. The less chance the toes have to encounter the front and top of the toebox, the less likely you are to bruise the nail beds.

If, despite your precautions, you become afflicted with black toenail(s), it is usually more of an esthetic than a medical problem. If you are a woman you can cover a black toenail with opaque nail polish. Or you can polish the unaffected ones black to match.

Overtraining

There are many stories of athletes whose performance, despite hard training, began to decline. The cure, they all thought, was to exercise still harder. Invariably, harder training worsened performance. As "long and hard" continued, a cascade of further unhappiness followed: the athletes became irritable and moody, their resting pulse rates rose, and they experienced insomnia and chronic fatigue. Even worse, lean body mass declined—a wasting phenomenon. In women athletes, long and hard training caused not only amenorrhea, but also a demineralization of bone. Young women exhibiting the overtraining syndrome had bones that resembled those of older women well beyond menopause.

These are the classic signs and symptoms of overtraining. The overtrained state and all its adverse chemistry is not easily reversed. Taking a day or even a week off from training does not change matters much; in severe cases, a rest of a few months is needed. Prevention is better. Here are the rules of prudence:

o Work out three or four days a week, not six or seven.
o Strong workouts should be about 45 minutes, or an hour at maximum.
o Keep your total weekly mileage well under 40.
o Be suspicious if performance starts falling off or resting pulse rate (taken in the morning) is ten beats higher than usual in the face of continued hard training.
o If you are exercising the day after a hard workout, ease up a bit on pace for that second day's workout. Exercising three or four days in a row is inadvisable unless every other day is an easy workout just for form.
o Balance intensity and distance. Longer workouts should be at a more moderate pace; shorter workouts can be stronger.

You will see and feel the rewards in a relatively short time. It is more important to make aerobic walking a part of your lifestyle, so that all the good metabolic things will continue forever.

Fire and Ice

Everyone knows that a very hot day or a very cold day can wipe you out in a single workout, even if you are careful to avoid overtraining and even if your muscles and bones are strong. The precautions to take against the extremes of hot and cold weather are mostly good common sense. Knowing the details of how the human body reacts to temperature variation gives you an extra edge in outwitting such environmental challenges.

Heat Injury. The main culprit in heat exhaustion or its extreme form, heat stroke, is not the sun or the ambient temperature of the air.

It is your own body's heat generation. You can collapse into uncon-
sciousness during a workout when the outside temperature is cooler
than your body temperature. A 93-degree-Fahrenheit day, for example, is pretty hot for exercising, but it is less than 98.6-degree-Fahren-
heit body temperature. Obviously, exercise stokes the engines of fire.

Our bodies ordinarily have good cooling mechanisms:

o Increasing respiratory rate and volume will cool by carrying
   away warm water vapor. It is a human panting reaction.
o We produce sweat which evaporates and cools us.
o Cooling occurs when we drink water to replace fluid losses.
o Direct heat exchange occurs when the outside temperature is
   lower than the body's surface temperature.

Sweating is a very efficient mechanism for cooling, but only if
the sweat evaporates. Transferring fluid from inside the skin to the
outside of the skin does not produce a transfer of energy. It is when
the sweat is transformed into a gaseous state upon evaporation that
the body is cooled. The rate of evaporation is inversely proportional
to the humidity of the air. When humidity approaches 100 percent,
the rate of evaporation approaches zero. Air at 85 degrees Fahrenheit feels like 85 degrees Fahrenheit when the humidity is 35 percent. If the humidity is 60 percent, 85 degrees feels like 90 degrees.
If the humidity is 90 percent, 85 degrees feels like 102 degrees. At
higher temperatures the effect of rising humidity produces larger
jumps in apparent temperature (Figure 22).

Certain individuals are more at risk than others exercising in
torrid temperatures. Children sweat less than adults and do not tolerate heat as well. The obese also do poorly in hot weather. So do the
unfit and those who are chronically dehydrated.

There are a few things you can do to reduce risk during summer workouts, other than sitting on a shaded patio with a cold gin
and tonic in your hand:

o Train well before the summer season. Aerobic fitness enables
   you to tolerate heat better, during both normal daily activities
   and exercise. An aerobically-trained body is more efficient at
   getting rid of the heat produced by its metabolic processes.

Actual Temperature: 85°F.

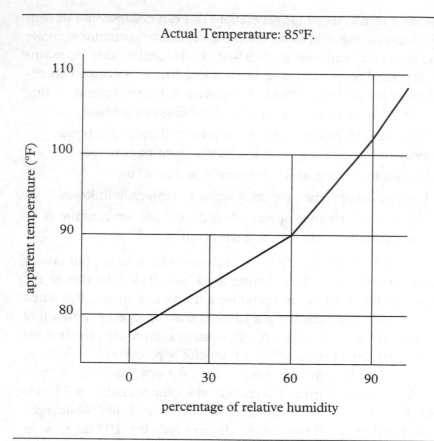

Figure 22.

o Wear light clothing that allows sweat to evaporate.

o Wear a hat that shades your face.

o Walk on shaded trails.

o Work out in the morning or evening rather than at midday. The danger hours on a hot, sunny day are 11 AM to 4 PM.

o Shorten and slow down your workout on a hot day.

o Drink generous amounts of water before, during, and after your workout. *The American College of Sports Medicine Position Stand on Prevention of Thermal Injuries during Distance Running* advises race directors to have water available every 2 to 3 km (1.2 to 1.8 miles) and advises athletes to drink 100 ml to 200 ml (3.2 oz to 6.4 oz) at each station. My own experience is that these recommendations are fine for temperatures up to 70 degrees Fahrenheit and moderate humidity. At 80 degrees Fahrenheit and/or higher humidity, I advise fluids every ½ mile. It is difficult to drink too much. You would have to drink gallons over the course of a few hours to overdo it. Water intoxication is so rare that only a couple of cases have been reported in the medical literature, and those are oddities.

o While you are taking water by mouth, it is a good idea to take a second cupful and pour it over your head.

o You can prepare yourself for a hot weather race by training to a high level of fitness and including some hot weather training in your workout schedule.

o Do not compete or do a hard workout if you are ill. Even a bad cold counts as illness.

o Know the early signs and symptoms of heat injury: loss of coordination, dizziness, nausea, headache, apathy, and either excessive sweating or lack of sweating.

o Have a partner who may be better able to evaluate your early signs.

o If you (or others) become aware of such an abnormal reaction, it is time to stop your workout immediately and get out of the sun. If the heat effect is more than mild and does not improve quickly when you stop, medical treatment is called for.

You do not have to give up your workouts for the entire summer. Just use good common sense and your new knowledge of how best to duel the heat.

Rules for Winter Workouts. Winter is not a valid excuse for four months of uninterrupted rest. You should not have to miss more than an occasional workout because of extreme weather conditions.

The following are the common winter problems, their practical solutions, and some matters that are beyond the pale.

o On slippery surfaces use a shorter stride and walk with well
   balanced posture. On snow, use shoes with heavy treads, even
   hiking boots. If the trail surface is icy, you may elect to sit indoors in front of a fireplace and do a mental imagery workout.

o Frostbite is a danger for exposed skin and for fingers and toes.
   Cover up in temperatures below freezing. Mittens are better
   than gloves, and there is no embarrassment in wearing a face
   mask. No one will recognize you in a mask.

o Hypothermia is a sort of core temperature frostbite. If the
   amount of heat you lose through your skin and breath is greater
   than the amount you generate by muscular work, your core
   temperature falls. At first you shiver; later a whole parade of
   more serious effects come marching through your body.
       The wind contributes to the cooling effect of cold air. The
   wind chill in cold weather is analogous to the temperature
   humidity index in hot weather. Both exaggerate the effect of
   temperature in a real way. Neither is an illusion.
       Hypothermia can occur at above-freezing temperatures as
   well. Rain at 35 degrees or 40 degrees Fahrenheit can be
   remarkably chilling because of the high specific heat of water.
   Cover every possible inch of bare skin to preserve heat. Your
   neck, especially, needs to be insulated because of the large blood
   vessels that are close to the surface. Proper clothing guards
   against both hypothermia and frostbite. The inner layer of cold
   weather clothing should allow the sweat to wick away from the
   skin. T-shirts and long johns made of polypropylene, or equivalent are best. The outer layer should be a windproof material
   such as nylon, dacron, or Gore-Tex™. Even when the air is at
   dead calm, you create a breeze of 4, 5, or 6 mph, depending on
   your walking speed. For the middle layer(s), wool is recommended. A hat to cover your head and ears, mittens or a pair of
   old wool socks for your hands, and a scarf or turtleneck gar-
   ment for your neck are all essential for retaining heat.

o No matter how you cover up, you still must breathe in air from
   the outside. When that air is less than 98.6 degrees Fahrenheit
   the body has mechanisms to make it more friendly to the lungs.

The nasal passages ordinarily warm and humidify the air we inhale so that the trachea (windpipe) and the passageways down into the lungs will receive body-temperature air. When the outside air is colder, it gets further down the respiratory airway before reaching body temperature. Air that is below freezing does not reach body temperature until it is well into the bronchi. The lining of the lower respiratory tract does not like cold, dry air and may complain about it.

What to do? You can continue to train in cold weather if you slow your pace a little and breathe in a more shallow fashion.

Winter can be a pleasant time to do outdoor workouts. The air is often clear and the sky vividly blue. The trails and byways are not as crowded with runners, cyclists, and skaters. The ozone levels are lower. We are not naturally hibernating creatures, and we continue our need for exercise. Go for it.

The Infernal Combustion Engine

As walkers we must deal with large variations in temperature and humidity. Our bodies usually adapt well, and we get enough air into our lungs to supply oxygen for aerobic workouts. Autos that share the nearby environment, though, can add significant amounts of carbon monoxide to the air we breathe. If there is any notable amount of carbon monoxide present, the oxygen-carrying hemoglobin of the red blood cells will be in trouble. Carbon monoxide, even in small concentrations, can be serious for athletes because it has an affinity for hemoglobin that is 1,000 times as great of that of oxygen. Carbon monoxide binds with hemoglobin to form carboxyhemoglobin (COHb), leaving no room on the molecule for oxygen. The working muscles, naturally, cannot do well when their supply of oxygen is limited.

Just as serious, a high level of carboxyhemoglobin reduces the availability of oxygen to the heart. High carboxyhemoglobin levels can produce:

1. Exercise-induced electrocardiogram changes that are typical of angina.

2. Disturbances in normal heart beat rhythms in people who have coronary heart disease . . . no exercise required.

Levels of carbon monoxide that can result in such athletic and medical problems are commonly found along urban roads and highways. A study from New York Hospital–Cornell University Medical Center, located in the midst of the fumes of Manhattan, measured levels of carboxyhemoglobin in runners in two locations—on the roadway in Central Park and along the F.D.R. Drive. The Central Park roadway is shared by pedestrians and autos during rush hours; the F.D.R. Drive and the adjacent East River footpath share air space at all hours. The COHb blood levels of the runners during exercise were high enough to cause cardiac abnormalities in anyone with coronary artery disease and probably some with normal hearts.

It is best to select workout sites well removed from traffic. Even Manhattan has places where cars cannot get through to threaten you physically or physiologically.

Be Street Wise

Walkers and runners travel light when they train. Logically, they do not make financially attractive victims. Women in athletic clothes who are moving fast should not make attractive victims either. But thieves and rapists are not logical. It is wise to follow some common sense rules of personal safety when working out.

o Be aware of your surroundings, especially the people. Be aware visually; be aware of the sound of footsteps; be aware with whatever sixth sense you may possess.

o Do not use head phones and tapes except where and when safety is assured.

o Be familiar with the course on which you are working out. Note surroundings such as shrubbery, open areas, places where you may get help if you are in trouble, such as public telephones, neighborhood shops, or a local tavern. Get to know the runners and walkers who regularly use the trail. A smile or "Good morning" to local residents is also a good idea.

o Do not work out in isolated areas or where the surroundings offer places of concealment for those who ask involuntary sharing of yourself or your belongings.

o Do not wear valuables openly.

o If your workout course is not well frequented, work out at different times of day. Some violence-prone individuals plan their attacks if they know you will be at a given place at a given time.

o If there is a questionable area you must pass on an otherwise safe course, plan your direction or starting/finishing point so you pass it early in the workout when you are fresher.

o Wearing a police-style whistle on a string is a deterrent to any would-be assailant. Blowing it is even more of a deterrent.

o Group workouts provide safety in numbers.

o Having a dog with sharp teeth as your walking partner upgrades the safety rating of any neighborhood. Violet, one of my walking students in Queens, has such a hound. When passing near anyone of questionable intent, she commands her companion, "Down, Duke, down!" No one suspects that Duke is only interested in making friends with the world.

o Keep an inviolate personal space of 10 or 12 feet around you. When anyone enters that personal space, reestablish your boundary distance immediately. If the individual closes in again, shout, "Get away!" Use obscenities if need be. Yell, "Rapist!" Blow your whistle. Do not be embarrassed. If the individual is really innocent of evil intent, it is he who should be embarrassed for having alarmed you.

o If you become trapped, you will have to use your best judgment as to whether to resist or not. There are many factors to consider: whether the assailant has a weapon, whether you are trained in self-defense, your size, the assailant's size, etc. Your best weapon may be the words you use. Many ploys are possible. You can suggest that you have a highly contagious disease.

Ask, "Does your mother know that you prey on innocent victims?" You can make gurgling, incomprehensible sounds followed by the facial contortions and body motions of a seizure
disorder. The possibilities are limited only by your imagination.

o Cyclists and rollerbladers generally have no antisocial intent.
But they pay little attention to traffic lights and stop signs. Play
it safe by looking both ways before crossing a road or pathway.

Aerobic walking is an inherently safe exercise. It can be even
more so with these simple precautions. Rather than walking on the
knife edge between safety and danger, keep a generous margin of
safety.

CHAPTER 11

Accessories
Outfitting for Aerobic Walking

Shoe Views

In the beginning there were shoes and there were sneakers. Then sneakers became specialized: for running, tennis, decks of cruise ships, and so on. Technology became sophisticated, and style, avant-garde. Special features were designed to provide cushioning, support, and stabilization. Then came gels and air, bubbles and tubes, flex zones and energy return systems, and finally it was psychedelic colors.

Technology was in fashion, and fashion said do not call them sneakers. So they became "shoes"—running shoes, tennis shoes, court shoes, cross-training shoes, and walking shoes.

Go into an athletic footwear shop these days and you will face a formidable array of brands and models. Do not be intimidated. Insist on trying on the sport-specific shoe of different manufacturers until you find a pair that suits the size and shape of your feet and your skill level.

The following tech specs focus on what to look for in the way of features.

Comfort. The shoe must be comfortable right at the start. It should feel as if it needs no breaking in. Each manufacturer makes its shoes on lasts that are supposed to have the configuration of the average American foot. I find it curious that, given this goal, no two shoe companies have the same lasts. But their lack of logic is your gain. You have many different "average" shapes to choose from and you are likely to find at least one that matches your feet. Try on a number of brands. Try on different models of each brand. Start with the walking shoes and the running shoes, and if none of those quite fits, try models designed for other sports.

Toe Room. The shoes should be roomy in the toe box, both laterally and vertically. There should be a little space in front of the toes as well. When trying on shoes, bring along the socks you will be wearing with the shoes in your workouts.

Flexibility. The shoe should flex at the ball of the foot where your foot flexes. Some shoes are too stiff, which inhibits a smooth, fluid stride. The shoe should not feel as if it has a plate of spring steel down its length. The spring of your own ligaments and tendons should not have to fight with the shoe.

Cushioning. As you increase the distance of each workout, you may be laying down as many as five or six thousand footsteps in 45 minutes. Your feet will appreciate the cushioning. Do not just take the shoe techie's word for it; put your hand in the shoe and press down on the insole. Put the shoes on your feet and walk around.

Heel Support. The heel counter should be firm because that is the part of the shoe you will pressing against as you spin the earth around backward with your powerful strides.

Achilles Notch. The uppermost part of the heel counter should dip down instead of ending in a high tab. If there is no Achilles notch, that upper edge will press into your own Achilles tendon at the end of each stride. A few hundred strides and your tendon will complain. It is better to prevent the problem at the start, in the shoe store (Figure 23).

Arch Support. The contour of the inside of the shoe should provide good arch support. The outer sole may rise a little to contribute to this support.

Getting a Grip. The bottom of the sole should have some amount of texture in the form of lines or patterns to provide traction, but should not have deep treads as in hiking boots. In walking, the swing

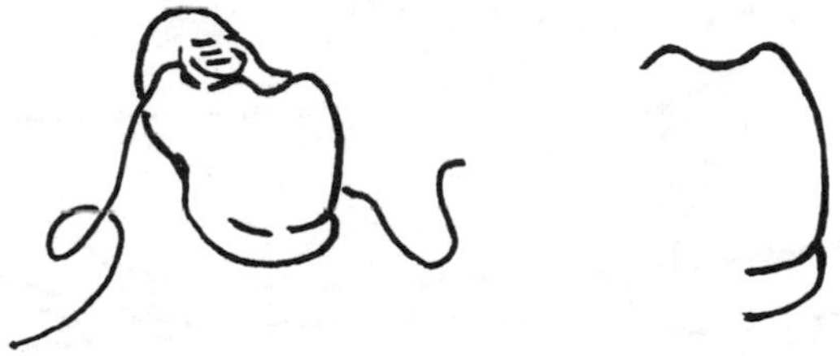

Figure 23. Achilles notch, rear view.

(or recovery) foot that comes forward for each next stride clears the ground by $\frac{1}{2}$ inch or less. Shoes with cleats and the like put you at risk of tripping. Leave the cleats to the hikers and runners.

Sole on a Roll. The profile of the sole should not be flat, but slightly convex. The shoe techies call this a rocker profile. It allows the foot to roll from the heel to the ball of the foot instead of slapping down at every stride (Figure 24).

Some running shoes have built up heels that, for walking, tend to tilt you too far forward. Walking shoes, and some of the low-tech running shoes, have heels that are more appropriate for walking.

Supple Uppers. When your foot bends, the upper of the shoe bends. If the material of the upper is too stiff, it can press into the top of the base of your toes. Uppers made of leather or imitation leather tend to be stiff. Nylon mesh is more pliable does not inflict the torture of a thousand steps.

Toe Tops. The one place on the upper of the shoe that needs heavier material is the spot that covers the end of the big toe. Walking technique requires the heel to contact the ground at a 30-degree to 40-degree angle. To achieve this angulation, the toes must press up

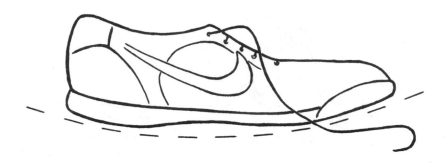

Figure 24.

against the upper of the shoe. Such pressure, repeated several thousand times each week, can wear right through lightweight uppers.

Nowadays, I do preventive maintenance on my shoes by gluing on a small oval of stiff material right over the big toe. I find that Shoe Goo®, used as cement, works well.

Ankle and Instep Padding. It is nice to have a padded collar and a padded tongue, though it is not an absolute necessity if you do not lace your shoes too tightly.

Heel Bevel. When you walk, the heel is the first part of your foot to contact the ground. The heel should not make contact on an edge but rather on a bit of a flat surface. A shoe with a 30-degree to 40-degree beveled heel will provide that flat surface. The bevel should not be so long that it extends far under the heel. In that case, you would slow down for an instant at heel contact (Figure 25).

These features are important in your choice of a shoe. The manufacturer may have other features, which can be considered a

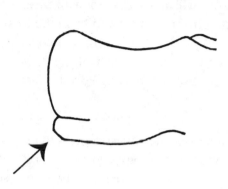

Figure 25. Heel bevel, side view.

luxury. Small perforations for air circulation and insoles that are removable for washing are nice if available in an otherwise good shoe. So is a small lacing loop on the top of the tongue to keep it from sliding left or right. Technologically well-designed shoes are easy to find. Shoes that fit well are more difficult to find.

When your technique becomes smoother and faster, you will probably prefer less cushioning and more flexibility. You will need a little less arch support. Fluid walking technique allows very gentle heel contact and no pounding. Technique, to some extent, replaces cushioning. Technique also establishes a sense of balance so there is less stress on the arch.

The energy-return capacity of human connective tissue, tendons in particular, can be over 90 percent. The materials used for the soles of shoes return less than 50 percent of the energy used to make them bend at every stride. Shoes that let the walker feel the ground and are very flexible allow the transfer of energy from muscles to tendons and into ground forces with little loss of power.

At first, athletic shoes were for athletes. Now, some women wear athletic shoes to their office and then change into heels for work. Traveling to the office in athletic shoes has several advantages: First is comfort. You will arrive at work with fresh feet. Second, dress shoes are protected from weather and from the wear and tear of foot travel over sidewalks, curbs, and manhole covers. Third, your feet are protected from the wear and tear of dress shoes. High heels can be your arch enemy. Fourth, walking speed is faster in athletic shoes.

Socks

It is hard for sports and fitness writers to become excited about socks. After all, what technology can be put into socks so that the wearer will set new world records? But there are some differences that you should know about.

o Cotton has the advantage of being inexpensive.

o Wool is warm.

o Polypropylene wicks out sweat.

o Nylon reinforces other materials.

o Two pairs of thin socks may be better than one pair of heavies, particularly for preventing blisters. The inner pair should be of polypropylene or an acrylic weave that breathes.

Sock manufacturers have not yet discovered that everyone has one right and one left foot; in every pair of socks, the two socks are identical. But you can outwit the manufacturer. After wearing a new pair of socks for the first time, each sock of the pair takes the shape of the foot it covered. Immediately label the socks R and L with a laundry marker, and you will have customized socks. Someday the sock manufacturers will follow the lead of the manufacturers of gloves and shoes and make a right and left in each pair.

Wear

The options of what to wear above the ankles are unlimited. The next-to-the-skin layer should breathe and not hold sweat in place. Polypropylene and special-weave polyester, such as Thermax® and CoolMax™ are best. Silk is okay, too.

If warmth is the goal, a good choice for the next layer is wool, which traps many tiny pockets of air. Wool is breathable and is actually as functional as polypro products. It is just that wool is much more itchy next to the skin.

The outer layer should be wind proof. Nylon keeps the wind out but also keeps the sweat in. An outer shell of a fabric such as Gore-Tex® has all the advantages except it is costly. Gore-Tex® is wind proof, water proof, and breathable. If your exchequer is in good shape, it is wonderful material for outerwear.

The above suggestions are the ideal, but they are not critical. Anything that is comfortable and works for you is fine. It is worth experimenting.

Hand Weights? Wait!

Walking has always been considered a minor exercise that induces only modest increases in fitness. One day, a bright entrepreneurial type decided that if walkers carried hand weights during their perambulations they would expend more energy and make walking into a more effective exercise.

A few studies have compared walking with and without hand weights. There is general agreement that swinging the hand weights vigorously while walking increases energy consumption at a given walking speed. Very neat, except no one stopped to think that one can walk faster without weights than with.

There is worse news. A study by J. E. Graves et al at the University of Florida reported a slight elevation in diastolic blood pressure and noted that "arm exercise involves a relatively small muscle mass that must develop a greater percentage of its maximal tension to perform a given amount of work." The authors theorize that there may be a compression of blood vessels that results in an increase in blood pressure. Other studies reported that systolic blood pressure also increases with the use of hand weights.

A simpler biomechanical problem with hand weights is the limitation on the rate of arm swing which, in turn, limits the rate of stride turnover and overall ground speed. A walker with hand weights walks more slowly than one without hand weights. The walker who moves faster without weights is using large, lower body muscles with greater vigor, which brings us back to the rule that a large muscle mass brings about a large metabolic change. It is better to put the effort into leg work. With good technique you can go fast enough to be right at aerobic/anaerobic threshold and burn calories to the max.

Another problem seen with hand weights is that the increased rotational force/momentum of each arm swing must be stopped and reversed at end-swing by the shoulder, chest, and back muscles. After a couple of thousand repetitions, these muscles may just give up in fatigue or go into spasm.

Further, good posture and balance are more difficult to maintain when using hand weights.

It all comes down to learning good walking technique with free hands.

Treadmills

When the weather turns your favorite trail into Class Five rapids, you may want to walk indoors. An indoor track is acceptable if you do not get dizzy on the tight curves. A shopping mall is fine if you can resist the inviting aromas of the pastry shop.

Another way in from the weather is to use a treadmill. Exercise physiologists like treadmills because pace is easier to measure, temperature and humidity are easier to control, and respiratory gases and cardiovascular dynamics, are easier to measure than when their subjects are running on an outdoor track. Early studies concluded that, in terms of oxygen consumption and energy expenditure, exercising on a treadmill was just as good as exercising outdoors on a track or trail. Only recently have some differences been found, especially in the measurement of perceived exertion.

I have found that it is easier to keep up with a treadmill belt that is doing the work than to spin the earth around backward with each stride. Raising the front of the treadmill three or four degrees seems to make it more the equivalent of Mother Earth.

Another difference I have noticed is that my sense of balance is disturbed for a minute or two when I step off the treadmill after a 45-minute workout. It is the same feeling as when coming ashore after a few days on a small sailing vessel. Whatever the explanation turn out to be, it adds weight to the argument that walking in place on a treadmill is different than walking a distance on the earth. I recommend Mother Earth whenever possible.

Walking Sticks

Walking sticks are probably as old as mankind. Humans have always walked. They walked when hunting and gathering food. They walked to find stones that could be chipped to fashion tools and weapons. They traversed uneven terrain and crossed streams. Some bright neolithic individual must have thought, "With a nice long stick, I can vault across that stream and not get my feet wet."

When animals were domesticated, shepherds found it handy to use a long crook to catch wayward sheep. They also found the crook to be a good walking stick on the hillsides and rocky pastures. In forests and trails, a sturdy walking stick also functioned as a staff for personal protection.

The rediscovery of walking in more recent years has prompted the sporting goods manufacturers to offer several models of walking sticks, including a top-of-the-line anodized aluminum, adjustable height, steel-tipped stick with a leather strap, priced at about 50 dollars.

Are walking sticks worthwhile? If you are hiking or just walking in the woods, a single walking stick is fun to use, but it would create stride asymmetry for workouts. Walking with a pair of poles, though symmetrical, limits stride speed and diverts work effort that should be concentrated in the lower body. Aerobic walking needs nothing but shoes and appropriate clothing.

Two of my octogenarian students used canes to get around when they first started walk training but soon improved to the point of not needing them. Yet, both continue to carry them for warning off automobiles when crossing streets.

For Women Only

Women runners not only have to worry about their knees, as male runners do, they have to deal with the force of stride impact on their breasts. Jogging bras are one solution. Aerobic walking is a better answer. Aerobic walking is kind to breasts, knees, and backs. The bounding motion of running has a vertical as well as a a horizontal vector. Aerobic walking, when well done, involves almost no up-and-down motion. Until you gain super fluid form, though, a sport bra is a good idea.

Sundries

If you like gadgets and gizmos, there are plenty of accessories to make you happy.

For carrying anything more than your house key, there are fanny packs, sling pouches, wrist pockets, and water-bottle holsters.

For keeping track of your time and distance, there are sports watches and pedometers. The digital timepieces track the time of your workouts accurately. The step counters count number of strides accurately, but when it comes to deducing distance, your stride length may vary during a workout and introduce error. I know that my stride in a four- or five-mile workout starts out at $3\frac{1}{2}$ feet per step. By the three-mile mark it dwindles to 3 feet, and with only 200 yards to go it approaches $3\frac{1}{2}$ feet per stride again. You can use the pedometer for fun or try to walk so smoothly that it does not register, but if you seriously want to measure distance, work out on a measured course. High school and college tracks are usually $\frac{1}{4}$ mile if they are old or 400 meters if they are new. For park trails, ask some of the runners who work out there. They know the distance of each loop to the tenth of a mile or closer. To settle a perennial distance dispute, the Central Park Reservoir track is 1.58 miles around.

For hot, sunny days, some kind of hat is advised. The varieties are endless. Hats can be a reflection of your persona, and nothing is too outrageous. It is your chance to walk on the wild side.

For night walking, it is best to be seen by motorists. Many manufacturers are using strips of reflective material on the sleeves and pants of their workout suits and on the heels of shoes. You can purchase reflective bands with velcro fasteners to wear around your arm. Reflective vests are also available—worn in the daytime you may get a friendly smile when passing road construction crews. Battery-powered flashing lights, one step ahead of reflectors in catching the eye of a motorist, are available in bicycle stores. They come with a strap meant to go around a handle bar but can just as well fit on a belt or on the strap of a fanny pack.

Headbands, whether for fashion or for keeping sweat from dripping down into your eyes, are made in many colors and patterns and messages. My own favorite has always been a paisley print kerchief rolled diagonally. I have them in six different colors to match or clash with different outfits.

After a strong, sweaty workout, most athletes like to take off their shoes and let their feet breathe. If you would like to treat your shoes as nicely, small bags of cedar chips are available to place inside for absorbing odors.

———————————

Any accessory, frivolous or vital, that makes you feel unique and raises your motivation level is all to the good. Do not deny yourself special things that add to your self-image as a walker.

CHAPTER 12

The Masters Class
The Fountain of Youth

When I lecture on the subject of aerobic walking as preventive medicine and tell audiences that they can be virtually as young as they
wish, the first thing they want to know is how old I am. I usually
invite them to participate in, or at least watch, a walk-training clinic
and decide for themselves.

Highly fit individuals who join the clinic discover that I move
effortlessly as I instruct them at a pace they find highly challenging.
They quickly realize that the question, "How old are you?" is not
answered by a simple number.

The Fountain of Youth

Age is a combination of medical/physical vitality, mental capacity, and emotional balance. None of these components is necessarily
related to how many times the earth has gone around the sun during your life.

High-quality exercise can make you young. Exercise bestows
the medical/physical status of a younger person. Exercise quickens
thought processing. Exercise creates resistance to both depression
and anxiety.

Have older Americans taken advantage of the magic of exercise? A few have, but how few is reflected in the health status of
senior citizens as a class. Half of all American men over the age of
65 have cardiovascular disease, most commonly coronary artery disease. Hypertension is rampant in both men and women past middle

age. Osteoporosis and loss of agility combine for record numbers of hip fractures. There is a 30 percent, or more, decline in work capacity from age 30 to age 70. Most individuals over 65 take prescription drugs for some medical problem.

The XYZ's of Aging

The loss of health and vigor with increasing years represents the final common pathway of decline of almost all the tissues of the body, the brain included. Here is a compendium of what usually happens as the years add up:

o   The size and strength of the muscles diminish.

o   The mineral content of the bones is reduced.

o   The heart muscle is less lean and strong.

o   The specialized heart tissues that initiate the electrical impulses causing the heart to contract are less certain in their rhythm.

o   The valves of the heart become thickened and less supple. No longer is there a free flow of blood from the upper to the lower chambers, to the lungs for aeration, and into the aorta for systemic circulation. Sometimes valve calcification occurs, making matters even worse.

o   The coronary arteries collect deposits on their inner surfaces, restricting the blood flow to the tissues of the heart, itself. Severe constriction is likely to result in angina; complete obstruction causes a heart attack.

o   The arteries of the systemic circulation become less elastic.

o   The capacity to utilize oxygen in the energy systems of the body is markedly reduced. This decline is a product of lower maximal heart rate, lower blood supply to the working muscles, and less oxidative activity in the cells' energy chemistry.

o   The control mechanisms of carbohydrate metabolism become less effective. The islet cells of the pancreas produce less insulin when the need arises, and the tissues of the body do not utilize the available insulin efficiently.

o   Secretion of the digestive enzymes declines.

o The kidneys are less efficient in regulating fluid balance and electrolytes (sodium, potassium, calcium, and others). There is a reduced filtration rate and a lessened capacity to conserve (re-absorb) water and sodium. Even thirst perception is dulled. The cardiovascular drugs that many seniors use generally worsen fluid and electrolyte balance.

o The complex immune system declines in function.

o The body's production of natural antioxidants is diminished, and there is a greater accumulation of free radicals that can damage cells.

o The body's biological rhythms become less synchronized. In younger individuals, the daily highs and lows of the body's production of different hormones and enzymes are well coordinated. As we age, daily rhythms such as sleep-wake cycles and sodium, chloride, and water excretion become more erratic.

o As we age, our mental processes are not as quick. Discrimination tasks and decision making are more difficult. Short-term memory is adversely affected. Many other parameters of brain function also decline with age.

We have all observed these changes associated with aging, in others if not in ourselves. Note that I said *associated with* and not *caused by* aging. Physiologists are now questioning whether the commonly seen changes are inevitable. Further, they are investigating whether such age-related changes can be reversed. We ought to think of the decline that accompanies aging as a deficiency disease that is properly treated with physical exercise.

Expect Better

Poets and playwrights, having more insight into the human condition, have long known of the preventive value of exercise. With uncommon wisdom they specified walking in their own exercise prescription (Smiley).

Emerson wrote: "To walk in the woods . . . is one of the secrets of dodging old age."

Dickens said: "The best way to lengthen out our days is to walk steadily and with a purpose. . . . Certain ancients, far gone in years, have staved off infirmities and dissolution by earnest walking—hale fellows, close upon ninety, but brisk as boys."

Physicians have long accepted the relationship between aging and physical and mental decline. The senior patients who come to their offices and clinics are usually there for the diagnosis and treatment of disease resulting from that decline. Many physicians estimate that half the decline is attributable to inactivity. My own view is that 50 percent is too conservative. I believe we can do more than merely slow down the rate of aging. If you have been inactive, you can *regain* a generous amount of your youth with exercise. Many of the declines seen with increasing age can be reversed. Thereafter, maintaining a high state of fitness permits only a very slow rate of decline in some facets of function. In others, there may be no decline at all for many more years.

Aging does not cause slowing down; slowing down causes aging.

In recent years a good deal of research has shown what exercise can do for the over-the-hill gang. The studies have investigated many facets of aging, and different approaches have been used to study the changes seen in the various systems (cardiovascular, respiratory, musculoskeletal, and so on) of exercising subjects. Confirmation has been plentiful. The following improvements were evident for all ages of exercising seniors, up to and including young nonagenarians:

o Muscle strength is improved greatly in men and women. Muscle size is increased only in men, Maria A. Fiatarone and her coworkers studied ten frail subjects living in a residence for the elderly in the Boston area and reported a 174 percent increase in strength after an eight-week exercise program of resistance training.

o Exercise training increases stamina and work capacity.

o The ability of the cardiovascular system to deliver oxygenated blood to the working muscles and the capacity of the muscles to use oxygen are improved by aerobic exercise. That improvement can be sustained for a surprising number of years by continued exercise.

Men and women in their seventies have shown up to a 40-percent increase in oxygen utilization capacity after as little as three months of training. One paper concluded that the oxygen utilization capacity of the muscle cells in competitive senior athletes is the same as in well conditioned young men, though not quite as high as in elite young athletes. There is now a general consensus that there is no age limit for starting an exercise program and no age limit for improving fitness.

o Exercise lowers both resting heart rate and activity heart rate at any given work level. At the same time, blood volume per heartbeat is increased.

o Blood pressure is normalized with aerobic exercise and kept normal with continued exercise. That stability can be maintained for decades.

In a long-term longitudinal study, blood pressures were recorded in a group of individuals who entered an exercise program in middle age. Those who continued to exercise had their blood pressure checked periodically over 23 years. Pressures, on average, were maintained at 120/78. In a sedentary control group of similar ages, average blood pressures increased to 150/90 over a comparable number of years. My own experience in instructing aerobic walking programs is that most hypertensive patients can bring their blood pressures down to normal a few weeks after reaching aerobic levels in walk training. Then, a great majority can use aerobic walking to maintain blood pressure in a narrow range of normal—forever.

o Improvement in calcium metabolism takes much longer, or at least much longer to measure. Within a year or two, however, different combinations of dietary calcium, exercise, and hormone replacement therapy produce increases in bone mineralization. Such increases have been reported in seniors of all ages up to 90 years. After bone density increases to a maximum for any individual, continued exercise reduces the usual one percent per year rate of decline to one-half percent or less.

Bone strength, of course, increases with greater bone density. But bone strength is also related to bone width and only exercise brings about both.

o Aerobic walking technique increases walking speed and agility. The Malkin Technique, which uses the hamstring and gluteal muscles, increases the tone and strength of these muscles. This increased muscle strength is especially important in preventing hip (neck of femur) fractures in seniors. There are normal tension stresses on the upper plate of bone in the neck of the femur as the weight of the upper body is supported on the legs. Conversely, there are compression forces on the lower plate. When the tension forces exceed the strength of the bone, as in a bad fall, a fracture results. Strong gluteal muscles can counter the tension stresses and prevent the fracture (Figure 26). Additionally, the agility, balance, and surefootedness that comes with aerobic walking can prevent the fall in the first place.

o The metabolic changes that occur with aerobic exercise are not limited to the body. Brain chemistry also changes. Several studies have documented such significant improvements in brain function that we must revise some of our conventional views on aging.

David E. Sherwood and Dennis J. Selder of San Diego State University recorded response time in discrimination and choice-making tests for subjects aged 23 to 59. Half the subjects were habitual runners; half were sedentary controls. Each group was further delineated by age (in decades). The non-exercising control group showed ever-slower response times from 20 to 29 years through 50 to 59 years. The runners, however, showed no significant differences in response times among the age groups. The 50- to 59-year- old runners were as quick thinking as the younger runners!

Robert E. Dustman and his coworkers at the Veterans Administration Medical Center of Salt Lake City, administered a neuropsychological test battery to a group of sedentary subjects, aged 55 to 70. The subjects were then divided into three groups. One underwent a four-month period of aerobic exercise training; the second had four

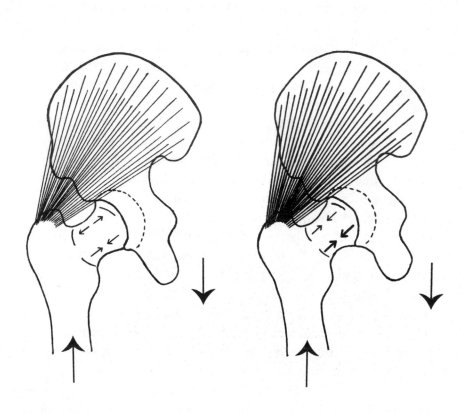

Figure 26. Rear view of hip joint and neck of femur strong gluteal muscles (right) counteract fracture causing tension forces at the upper plate of the neck of the femur.

months of strength and flexibility training; and the third was a sedentary control group. After the four-month trial, the test battery was administered again. The aerobic exercise group demonstrated substantial improvement in visual organization, mental flexibility, response time, and other measures of cognitive (thought processing) function. The group trained in strength and flexibility showed considerably less improvement, and the sedentary controls, none at all.

Louise Clarkson-Smith and Alan A. Hartley at Scripps College, in Claremont, California reported that a group of 62 men and women, aged 55 to 88, who were habitual exercisers, performed significantly better on measures of reasoning, working memory, and response time than 62 nonexercising controls in the same age range. Rita Friedman and Ruth M. Tappen of the University of Miami School of Nursing studied patients with Alzheimer's disease and reported improved communication performance among those in an exercise walking group and no improvement in a control group who participated in conversation sessions.

With the realization that wellness programs are the best answer to health care reform and with the discovery that exercise can bring about remarkable health improvements in the elderly, we are likely to see an increasing number of studies with senior citizens as subjects.

Possible and Impossible

The question of whether the elderly are capable of exercising at high enough levels of distance and intensity to achieve improvement in fitness has been answered by many studies showing significant gains in septuagenarians, octogenarians, and even nonagenarians.

Yet, the medical establishment considers exercise only an adjunct to drug therapy in the treatment of hypertension, diabetes, coronary artery disease, obesity, and other chronic diseases.

The A.M.A. Council on Scientific Affairs advised in its report, *Exercise Programs for the Elderly*, that, "when the physician finds no reason to exclude physical activity he [or she] should formulate an individualized exercise recommendation." Elsewhere the report suggests that walking "is a rhythmic activity suitable for older persons, placing minimum stress on the heart."

In a report published in the journal, *Primary Cardiology*, Drs. D. D. Schocken and J. A. Blumenthal acknowledge that "physical conditioning should be a fundamental part of the overall management of elderly patients." But they "strongly advise against overzealousness" in prescribing exercise.

It is true that seniors who are sedentary need to progress more gradually in their exercise program than young professional athletes, but they are capable of reaching high fitness levels. They may even become competitive athletes. The Masters Sports Program under The Athletic Congress (successor to the A.A.U.) includes several different sports, most notably, track and field. The achievements of some of these athletes in every age category is astounding: a 60-year-old miler clocked at under 5 minutes, a 65-year-old pole vaulter clearing 12' 4", a 64-year-old racewalker averaging 8¼ minutes per mile for 3.1 miles (5 km). Amazing records have been set in every other event as well. These are not rare individuals with superhuman skills. Master athletes number in the thousands across the nation, and while they all do not set age-graded world records, almost all of them are turning out physical performances ordinarily expected of much younger individuals.

A few athletes have not been content to compete in their own age group. They have tested their skills against the best in the world in open competition. In professional sports, Nolan Ryan was still striking out Major League batters at age 46. Satchel Paige, the age-less pitcher, was winning games for the Cleveland Indians in 1965 at his official age of 59—everyone knew he was really past 60. Jack Nicholas won the Masters Golf Classic in Atlanta (open to all ages) when he was 46. Seven years later at age 53, he was tied for the lead after the first round with a 5-under-par 67. Arnold Palmer, competing at age 63, birdied the first three holes that year.

In dance, an athletic discipline as demanding as any of the professional sports, Edward Villella at age 53 performed in *Watermill* with even more grace and invention than he had eleven years earlier in his last previous performance.

An example of a good but not extraordinary athlete who keeps young is Laura, one of the guests at the health spa where I have taught aerobic walking. Laura, who is in her early fifties, has arranged her life around the central theme of fitness. Regular workouts, stretch sessions, and free-weight training are integral to her lifestyle. Another guest, Stanley, is a 29-year-old runner who does road work regularly in preparation for races sponsored by the New

York Road Runners Club. He has completed many races from 5 K to marathons. Stanley estimates his state of fitness as fairly high.

The fitness test that I administered at the spa was a timed, one-mile walk on a local high school track. The time recorded for each individual was age-rated and compared to time ranges on a chart of fitness levels. (See figure 5.)

Laura's time was 12 minutes flat. Stanley's was 11 minutes 20 seconds. That difference is very small in view of their 20-plus age difference. I would venture that Laura's one-mile walk time when she was 29 was likely close to Stanley's present time, which would mean that her level of fitness has hardly declined in over 20 years.

Fitness as measured by a one-mile walk test or by maximum oxygen capacity may be an exercise physiologist's way of measuring age-related decline, but you can use measures more relevant to daily living. Do you get tired after shoveling snow from the front walk? Are you out of breath climbing three flights of stairs when the elevator is out of order? Are you afraid you will not make it back after hiking five miles out on a woods trail? Such are the measures that can be returned to the high levels of your youth. All it takes is walking every other day. Technique (chapter 3) and how far, how fast, how often (chapter 4) will do the rest.

The final line on possibilities as a result of regular walking comes from the studies of the centenarians in different parts of the world. In these cultures individuals commonly live to the number of years that was allotted to Moses. More importantly, they live vital lives to the end of their days. Many studies have attempted to find their secret. Various hypotheses—yogurt, wine, minerals in the drinking water, and they like—have been proposed; but few investigators have given serious consideration to one particular common denominator of all these cultures: extensive walking. I hereby propose walking for inclusion on the left side of the equation whose right side reads "long lived and lively."

We do not have high valleys and plateaus to walk as the Hunzas and Abkhasians do, but we have parks and quiet neighborhoods.

We cannot completely avoid automobiles as they do, but we can minimize our contact with the infernal machines. We can walk for transportation when possible, and we can walk for exercise. We can try to keep our body's chemical plant humming smoothly and we can test the limits of the human life span.

CHAPTER 13

Small Miracles
Blessings Left and Right

In terms of what is possible for health and weight loss, there are no miracles, despite the above title. High levels of health are *routinely* achieved with aerobic walking, and chronic diseases such as hypertension, coronary artery disease, and osteoporosis are actually reversed. Exercise-induced health occurs practically every time. Yet, if some examples of health and shapeliness inspire us, we may count them as small miracles.

The health miracles reported in the popular magazines are usually instantaneous—going to a shrine on crutches and leaving without them, having sight restored by laying on of hands, to name just two. The miracles that come with aerobic walking are a little slower, but far more common. The following are a sampling from my personal experience over a period of eight years and illustrate that such miracles are available to anyone.

Eugenia Zuckerman, the renowned flutist, is a serious walker and works out regularly, regardless of weather. Ms. Zuckerman is not only a world class flutist, she is a writer and a TV arts correspondent. She says her walking workouts clear her head of mental toxins, and she then gets the best ideas for her fiction writing. She does her workouts the first thing in the morning and feels that the exercise kick-starts her metabolism for the day. When I asked her if the aerobic walking helped her flute playing, she replied, "Of course. You need the lung power for any wind instrument." Her answer was very matter-of-fact, as if endurance exercise were a requirement for all flutists.

Eugenia does not consider the benefits of aerobic walking to be miraculous. In her case, I disagree. She and Anthony Newman recently presented a series of three concerts at the New York Public Library. She acted as historian and lecturer as well as musician, presenting the social and political perspectives of the time in which the composers lived. She played each piece so effortlessly it almost seemed as if entire movements were played on a single breath. At the end of each piece, the applause lasted 15 or 20 seconds. She immediately introduced the next piece, speaking as easily as she had just played. To give you an idea of the final program's degree of difficulty, the artists performed sonatas by Marcello, Sammartini, Scarlatti, and Locatelli, and finished with the technically difficult Vivaldi *Sonata in A Major.*

I do not know whether 20 percent or 80 percent of Eugenia's respiratory reserve can be attributed to aerobic walking, but I do know that her performance was miraculous.

Nancy T. is a fitness person. She enjoys food and relies on exercise to keep shapely. She had been doing high-impact "aerobics" four times a week when she asked me about aerobic walking. She and her husband were thinking about starting a family and she wanted an exercise that would avoid the bouncing. We arranged a mini-course, and Nancy learned the technique nicely. Not yet pregnant, she continued to do high-impact aerobics but did add a walking workout one or two days a week.

When she became pregnant it was an easy switch to all aerobic walking. Nancy continued walking three to four times a week, and for seven months she did not look pregnant. At 30 weeks, she had gained 15 pounds and felt wonderful. At 35 weeks, she was still moving around the office where she worked faster than anyone else.

Nancy's blessed event time came early according to her calculations. Her membranes broke while driving home from a visit with friends. She called her obstetrician who instructed her to rest at home overnight but to call if contractions started. Seven hours later at 4 AM she was in the hospital and in labor. Nancy worked in labor for two hours without drugs or anesthesia and delivered a healthy baby girl who announced her presence in a loud, clear voice. Nancy opined that the muscles she used for birthing her child were strong from walk training. Most of her friends say that Nancy's labor and delivery were miraculously easy. Nancy says any woman can do it.

Malcolm McKesson is a painter who exhibits regularly in New York City. When I met him he was working primarily in pen, brush, and ink, and he carried the tools of his trade with him everywhere. Manhattan's wondrous old architecture fascinated him, and he was out at all hours of the day to find buildings and cityscapes in the most advantageous light.

Malcolm, at 84 years of age, suffered from a variety of leg and back ailments. When he began to have serious trouble in getting around to pursue his calling, a friend who knew of my work asked me to speak with him. The three of us met and discussed the possible advantages of aerobic walking for his infirmities. I suggested that the smooth walking technique I teach would probably reduce the pressure on his joints and ease his knee pain. A second scenario was that he would improve the circulation to his legs. We agreed to a first lesson.

When I arrived on the appointed day, Malcolm was wearing an orthotic in one shoe, had a lower leg wrapped in bandages, was wearing a knee brace and a back brace. Well!

I asked why the coach and the general manager of his team did not provide better offensive linemen to protect their starting quarterback. Malcolm laughed, and we discussed the specific reasons for each of the orthopedic aids. I explained the rationale for the technique used in aerobic walking and demonstrated the proper form. Then, we were off to Madison Square Park for our lesson.

Over the next four weeks, Malcolm and I worked on smoothness of form, better posture, and raising endurance levels. By the end of the month he had substantially copied my form, and found no further need for any of the artifices. He also increased his walking speed and agility.

Malcolm has continued to work out on his own and easily walks two or three miles if that is where an interesting building or fountain awaits his talents.

Nina K. was one of my health spa walkers. She had but two classes the first weekend I met her and was able to pick up only a few of the basics of technique. Her motivation, though, leaped ahead of her physical skills, and she became an avid walker.

Later that year, our paths crossed again at the spa. She came over to my table the evening that I arrived and had a bemused, self-confident look about her. "Hi Mort. I have news for you; I stopped smoking."

"Good for you," I replied.

"I'm not sure you understand. It was the walking—your walking," she insisted.

Nina went on to tell me how many times, over how many years, she had tried to stop smoking. She did it this time by extensive walking. Aerobic walk training gave her the endurance to walk for hours at a time. She had no nicotine craving and felt no anxiety. Now Nina walks only for an hour, three or four times a week, and she is the sole owner of her body and brain.

As a point of physiological interest for me, she said she could finally take a deep breath of fresh air. It seems that smokers can not breath deeply except when inhaling on a cigarette. This time Nina knew she was free forever.

Joyce Y. is another of the spa's guests who has taken to walking. She still jogs a little and bikes, but feels that aerobic walking has added another dimension to her overall state of fitness. She says that walking adds variety and has given her a greater tolerance for heat and cold. That tolerance has had some nice fallout at the United Nations agency where she works.

Joyce is soft spoken in both her personal and professional life. Although her views have always been respected, she has never been a dominant voice at the staff meetings of her agency. A few months after adding aerobic walking to her exercise mix, a strategic planning meeting was scheduled at which all 60 staff members were to be present. The meeting was held in a newly opened solarium that had large glass doors to an outdoor patio. It was a brisk fall day, and, even with the glass doors closed, the room temperature was on the cool side. As the meeting started, the participants, one by one, rose to get jackets or sweaters. Joyce just sat there in her thin cotton blouse and slacks, perfectly comfortable. The others took note, and, as the discussions continued, they looked to Joyce for leadership.

She told me, in recounting the meeting, "I like being tough without having to shout."

Small miracles also occur across the East River in Brooklyn. Joyce K. and I live a few blocks apart, and she had occasionally seen me moving fast on the way to the subway. When I started a small walking group in the neighborhood, she joined the gang partly out of curiosity.

In my preliminary lecture/demonstration, I mentioned that with aerobic walking, diligents could expect to reduce hypertension, stabilize blood sugar, and reduce cardiac risk factors. Those in the group who had any medical problems were advised to discuss the graduated walking program with their physician.

Joyce thought to herself, "If this kind of walking helps the heart, why wouldn't it help the lungs, too?" Although she was asthmatic, took medication regularly, and was limited in her daily activities, her physician felt she would benefit from regular walking. We decided on a nice, steady—but slow—rate of progress.

Over the next few months, Joyce gradually worked up to 60-minute workouts which she did three or four times a week at a good pace. Nice, but not astounding—not the world class levels a few asthmatics have reached in other sports. In a recent interview, Joyce told me that her miracles were more every-day in nature:

o She was able to reduce her asthma medications by more than half.

o She lost weight and size and now has a waistline that she had not known for years.

o She became more agile and gained stamina.

o She finally stopped smoking for good and has had no nicotine craving.

What was an asthmatic doing smoking? Joyce both asked and answered the question. She said that for years she had smoked close to a pack a day. As her asthma became worse she cut down to eight or ten cigarettes a day.

"You know, when I was having a cup of coffee or talking on the phone, it was easy to light up." she explained. "Now, it is easy not to smoke. In fact, if someone else is smoking and I can smell it, I feel sick."

Did Joyce's asthma improve because of her workouts or her smoke-out? Probably, both. We have seen in recent years that a number of diseases—diabetes, coronary artery disease, osteoporosis, and others—have multiple risk factors and respond best to a compendium of lifestyle improvements. Asthma, like these chronic diseases, involves more than one factor, and it pays to get all the help you can.

David L. also has asthma. His business takes him into Manhattan frequently, and frequently the air in Manhattan is less than fresh and clear. Because he usually makes several stops, he walks from one appointment to another. In past years David has often had to slow down his frenetic pace or even stop for a "breather" in an air-conditioned restaurant. Like other asthmatics, he could sense when continued effort would get him in trouble.

I first learned that David was asthmatic two years ago when he was hospitalized with an acute attack. After he was stabilized and returned home, we embarked on a graduated walking program. The first day's workout was a slow ten minutes. We added a few minutes every week or two and he easily achieved 40 minutes at a brisk pace. It is now two years since that first session, and he does 30- to 40-minute workouts regularly. These days, he easily completes a schedule of appointments that two years ago might have precipitated an attack. He says he no longer feels at risk. He is still careful about days with high pollen counts and still aware that he has asthma, but he does not feel like the disabled person he was two years ago. It is a small miracle.

Violet C. has always considered herself healthy. She is recently retired from teaching and was pleased to have the time to enjoy a leisurely breakfast each morning, to take an afternoon art class, and generally to be free of tight schedules. Her daughter, who knew of my work, had been after Violet to take walking lessons. After several weeks of being badgered, she found it easier to call me than to put up with her daughter's relentless reminders.

"Hello, this is Violet C. My daughter, Denise, said I should call you about walking lessons. Can you tell me what kind of walking you teach?"

It was not going to matter how I answered her question. Her children had increasingly been reminding Violet to stop dragging her feet, and she figured that walk lessons might help her to walk lightly. If no improvement occurred, she could at least say she put forth her best efforts. Then everyone would get off her case.

When I arrived for the first lesson, I found a 69-year-old woman, slightly heavy-set, who walked with clumpy footsteps. She said she was in good health and, indeed, ran her household capably. After explaining the form I would teach and the rationale for it, we went out for a warmup and a ten-minute "workout." The lesson was as much for me to discern her musculoskeletal needs as it was for her to improve her gait. Over the following weeks, Violet learned more about aerobic walking form and made gradual gains in endurance, pace, and self-confidence. In a period of a few months— lessons plus homework-workouts between the lessons—Violet could walk 50 minutes at a strong pace. Then the miracles began.

It is more vivid to compare the pre-walk-trained Violet with the new person afterward. She recently agreed to make a list of changes that she felt she could attribute to aerobic walking.
Here is her pre-walking list.

o Walked in a halting fashion with heavy footsteps

o Was in constant fear of tripping on a twig or uneven pavement

o When walking with another person (most often one of her adult children), would hold the other person's arm

o Pain in her feet when walking

o Knee pain when descending stairs

o Back pain when carrying a bag of groceries

o Wrapped toes and feet in lambs wool and placed foam rubber "spacers" between the toes

o Wore orthotics in both shoes
o Experienced swelling of the left leg at the end of the day
o Spent most of the day indoors; TV sets were on most of the time
o Felt weary every day from mid to late afternoon
o Bundled up with heavy clothing in winter, and wore slacks, never shorts, in summer

Here is Violet's since-walking list.

o Can walk for an hour at a brisk pace
o When coming upon a twig or small stone, can kick it without losing a stride
o Can actually run for 100 yards
o Never takes the arm of a companion when walking (In fact, her children have learned not to offer an arm anymore.)
o Uses no orthotics, lambs wool, or Band-Aids for feet and toes
o Feet do not hurt when walking
o Knees do not hurt when going up and down stairs (and nowadays she moves pretty fast both up and down)
o Leg no longer swells
o Does not watch TV during the day—unless the Mets are playing
o Explores around her neighborhood, delighting in discovering a working farm about a mile from home, finding a new trail in a nearby park, and retracing the route her children used when they walked to grade school many years before
o If the day is dark and cloudy, or even if it is drizzling, goes out to challenge the weather gods
o Tolerates cold better
o Keeps the thermostat at a lower temperature and does not bundle up excessively in winter
o Has grown perfect fingernails for the first time in many years

Violet feels that walking has created a whole new life for her. What I have seen is only better balance, much faster walking speed, far greater stamina, more self-confidence, and a brighter outlook.

She is also more attentive to her general surroundings as she walks instead of worrying about where to place each footstep. But if Violet thinks it is miraculous, it is miraculous.

Zelma is a small lady in height but a large woman in circumference. When she started in the walking program that I introduced to northeastern Pennsylvania, her measurements were as follows: chest = $42\frac{1}{2}$", waist = $43\frac{1}{2}$", and hips = $53\frac{1}{2}$".

One of her goals was to reduce her waist size to $42\frac{1}{2}$" so that it would no longer be larger than her chest size. Another was to curb her appetite and lose weight.

She took her measurements again after five weeks of aerobic walking, the first three weeks of which were not yet at aerobic threshold distance or pace. Thus, the results represent only two weeks at threshold levels. Her measurements after five weeks were as follows: chest = $41\frac{1}{2}$", waist = $42\frac{1}{2}$", hips = $52\frac{1}{2}$".

Zelma achieved her initial goal of a $42\frac{1}{2}$" waist, but because her chest also became smaller she did not attain the one-to-one chest/waist ratio. Still, she was more than happy to lose an inch in each dimension. She also listed several other positive results.

"I have more energy. I lost four pounds. My appetite is easier to control. I have tighter buns. I am happier, and my sense of humor has improved."

Then she had a complaint. "But my memory hasn't improved that much." Zelma, I only promised *small* miracles.

Dr. Marcellus Walker, her physician who was responsible for bringing the walking program into being, recently told me that Zelma has continued to walk regularly. I am scheduled to present another walking program for his patients soon and can not wait to see Zelma's chest/waist ratio and to see how smooth and fast she has become.

Abby D. has many professional letters after her name—RN, BSN, MSN, and ANP. She supported herself through graduate school by doing hospital bedside nursing a couple of evenings a week and on occasional weekends. She remembers that in her last four grueling years she had no time for exercise.

Her first regular job as a nurse practitioner was in hospice-home care. She was responsible for visiting patients and families at their homes, so that she could minister to their needs in their most familiar surroundings. She usually had to travel by subway, and her patients often lived in walk-up tenement apartments, sometimes on the fourth or fifth floor. Abby discovered on the very first day that climbing subway stairs caused shortness of breath; and when it came to a fifth floor walk-up, she had to stop and rest every two flights. She says that by the fifth floor, her patients had to resuscitate her. She was in a quandary and seriously questioned whether she would be able to keep the job for long. She felt unhappy about her own fitness level, and she also felt she was letting her patients down by being a poor role model for the healthful lifestyle that she was teaching. Being overweight and chronically tired, she felt more like a patient, herself.

About two months after starting her job, she saw a notice for a racewalking course at a nearby Y. She quickly signed up and hoped this would be the miracle she needed. Abby says that she is not athletic and had to put some concentrated effort into learning the form for racewalking. But that was easy compared to the graduate work she had recently completed.

For the first month of the walking course, Abby worked out three to four times a week and increased her distance from 20 minutes slowly to more than 30 minutes briskly. She began to find the workouts less an unpleasant duty and more an invigorating exercise. And, miracle of miracles, she found it easier to climb subway stairs and tenement flights. After another two months of regular walking, she lost inches, gained further stamina, and reduced her resting heart rate from 80 to 68. She also came to realize how precious her own life is and began to enjoy it more.

This last was no small miracle.

Marsha C. has always worked out regularly, using different exercise routines. One of her favorite sports is volleyball. With all that physical activity, why did she sign up for a walking course? I am not sure she, herself, really knew why. Perhaps it was some subconscious proprioceptive sense that told her that she had still higher potential. The six instructed sessions extended over a period of eight weeks. At the last session Marsha asked when the next course would be held. She was asking mostly for her friends who saw changes in her that they wanted for themselves. Marsha had become more self-confident, improved her posture from good to excellent, moved more easily, and became energized. That is what her friends saw. Marsha, herself, was more excited about the improvement in her volleyball playing.

"Now I'm like a leopard on the court. Nothing gets by me, and I ace anything near the net."

Marsha gained an awareness of her body and learned how to have it do her bidding. She feels that her walking workouts have changed her life—a small miracle. I say she was always capable of being what she has become.

The above small miracles and the few mentioned in earlier chapters are only a sampling. You, too, may find changes that you never expected, and whichever ones come to pass will be valuable. Aerobic walking can accentuate the positive in everyone.

REFERENCES

Allen, D. B., and M. J. MacDonald. "Post-exercise Late-onset Hypoglycemia." *Cardiovascular Reviews & Reports* 9 (1988): 60–62.

American College of Sports Medicine. "Position Stand on Prevention of Thermal Injuries during Distance Running." *Medicine and Science in Sports and Exercise* 16 (1984): ix–xiv.

Applegate, L. "Get the Fat Out: Fifty Tips to Lean Eating for Better Performance and Health." *Runners' World* (July 1991): 53–87.

Aprill, D. "Snowshoeing—the Other Winter Sport." *The Conservationist* 45 (1991): 16–21.

Bandura, A. "Behavioral Psychotherapy." In *Readings From Scientific American, Contemporary Psychology,* 387–394. San Francisco: W. H. Freeman, 1971.

Barnard, R. J., G. W. Gardner, et al. "Cardiovascular Responses to Sudden Stress Exercise—Heart Rate, Blood Pressure, and ECG." *Journal of Applied Physiology* 34 (1973): 833–837.

Barnard, R. J., R. MacAlpin, et al. "Ischemic Response to Sudden Strenuous Exercise in Men." *Circulation* 48 (1973): 936–942.

Beardsley, T. "The A team: Vitamin A and Its Cousins are Potent Regulators of Cells." *Scientific American* (February 1991): 16, 19.

Behen, M. "Tuber or Not Tuber: the Roots of Nutrition." *American Health* (March 1988): 121–130.

Berscheid, E., E. Walster, and G. Bohrnstedt. "Body Image." *Psychology Today* (November 1973): 119–131.

Bhambhani, Y. N., and M. Singh. "Metabolic and Cinematographic Analysis of Walking and Running in Men and Women." *Medicine and Science in Sports and Exercise* 17 (1985): 131–137.

Bhambhani, Y. N., P. Eriksson, and P. S. Gomes. "Transfer Effects of Endurance Training with the Arms and Legs." *Medicine and Science in Sports and Exercise* 23 (1991): 1035–1041.

Black, J. S., and W. Kapoor. "Health Promotion and Disease Prevention in Older People: Our Current State of Ignorance." *Journal of the American Geriatric Society* 38 (1990): 168–172.

Bogardus, C., S. Lillioja, et al. "Familial Dependence of the Resting Metabolic Rate." *New England Journal of Medicine* 315 (1986): 96–100.

Bouchard, C. "Genetic Factors in Obesity." *Medical Clinics of North America* 73 (1989) 67–80.

————. "Heredity and the Path to Overweight and Obesity." *Medicine and Science in Sports and Exercise* 23 (1991): 285–291.

Bouchard, C., A. Tremblay, et al. "Genetic Effect in Resting and Exercise Metabolic Rates." *Metabolism* 38 (1989): 364–370.

————. "The Response to Long-term Overfeeding in Identical Twins." *New England Journal of Medicine* 322 (1990): 1477–1482.

Brehm, B.A. "Standing-tall Fitness: the Posture Component." *Fitness Management* (June 1991): 30.

Breslin, J. "She's Still Our Sweetheart." *New York Newsday* (15 September 1991): NY4.

Brock, M. A. "Chronology and Aging." *Journal of the American Geriatric Society* 39 (1991): 74–91.

Brown, M. D. "Low back Pain and Sciatica—Conservative Treatment that Helps Most Patients." *Consultant* 31 (1991): 36–39.

Brownell, K. "The Yo Yo Trap." *American Health* (March 1988): 78–84.

Brownell, K. D., and S. N. Steen. "Modern Methods for Weight Control: the Physiology and Psychology of Dieting. *The Physician and Sportsmedicine* 15 (1987): 122–137.

Bruce, R. A. "Exercise, Functional Aerobic Capacity, and Aging—Another Viewpoint." *Medicine and Science in Sports and Exercise* 16 (1984): 8–13.

Brunt, D., and E. J. Protas. "Contribution of the Stance and Swing Limb to the Kinetics of Gait Initiation." *Medicine and Science in Sports and Exercise* 23 (1991): S–8.

Bursztyn, M., M. Bresnahan, et al. "Effect of Aging on Vasopressin, Catecholamines, and Alpha 2-Adrenergic Receptors." *Journal of the American Geriatric Society* 38 (1990): 628–632.

Busse, M. W,. and N. Maessen. "Effect of Consecutive Exercise Bouts on Plasma Potassium Concentration during Exercise and Recovery." *Medicine and Science in Sports and Exercise* 21 (1989): 489–493.

Campaigne, B. N. "Body Fat Distribution in Females: Metabolic Consequences and Implications for Weight Loss." *Medicine and Science in Sports and Exercise* 22 (1990): 291–296.

Caranasos, G. J., and R. Israel. "Gait Disorders in the Elderly." *Hospital Practice* 26 (1991): 67–94.

Carek, P. J., and T. C. Namey. "Include Exercise in Treatment for Anxiety." *Your Patient and Fitness* 6 (1992): 10–18.

Casaburi, R., and K. Wasseman. "Exercise Training in Pulmonary Rehabilitation." *New England Journal of Medicine* 314 (1986): 1504–1511.

Cavagnaro, D. A. "New Zealand." *Walking Magazine* 2 (1987): 18–22.

Ceci, R., and P. Hassmen. "Self Monitored Exercise at Three Different RPE Intensities in Treadmill vs. Field Running." *Medicine and Science in Sports and Exercise* 23 (1991): 732–738.

Cefalu, W. T. "Diabetes Management: No Man Is an Island." *Modern Medicine* 58 (1990): 10.

Center for Science in the Public Interest. "Eaters' Digest: Nutrition and Nuts." *Nutrition Action Health Letter* 13 (1986): 11.

Chazen, J. A. "Aluminum in Bone in Diabetic Patients." *New England Journal of Medicine* 317 (1987): 386.

Chodzko-Zajko W. J., and R. L. Ringel. "Physiological Fitness Measures and Sensory and Motor Performance in Aging." *Experimental Gerontology* 22 (1987): 317–328.

Clark, N. "How to Pack a Meatless Diet Full of Nutrients." *The Physician and Sportsmedicine* 19 (1991): 31–34.

———. "Milk: Destroying the Myths." *The Physician and Sportsmedicine* 18 (1990): 133–135.

Clarkson-Smith, L., and A. A. Hartley. "Relationships between Physical Exercise and Cognitive Abilities in Older Adults." *Psychology and Aging* 4 (1989): 183–189.

Cohen, J. A., and K. F. Gross. "Peripheral Neuropathy: Causes and Management in the Elderly." *Geriatrics* 45 (1990): 21–34.

Consumer Reports. "These Shoes Are Made for Walking." (February 1990): 88–93.

Consumer Reports. "Are You Eating Right?" 57 (1992): 644–655.

Cook, T. C., R. E. LaPorte, et al. "Chronic Low Level Physical Activity as a Determinant of High Density Lipoprotein Cholesterol and Subfractions." *Medicine and Science in Sports and Exercise* 18 (1986): 653–657.

Costill, D. L., M. G. Flynn, et al. "Effects of Repeated Days of Intensified Training on Muscle Glycogen and Swimming Performance." *Medicine and Science in Sports and Exercise* 20 (1988): 249–254.

Council on Scientific Affairs. "Exercise Programs for the Elderly." *Journal of the American Medical Association* 252 (1984): 544–546.

Country Inn Collection. *New England's Finest Country Inns.* Toll-free telephone number: 1-800-852-4667.

Cowan, M. M., and L. W. Gregory. "Responses of Pre- and Post-menopausal Females to Aerobic Conditioning." *Medicine and Science in Sports and Exercise* 17 (1985): 138–143.

Cremons, A. N. "Minimizing Injuries in Habitual Runners." *The Physician and Sportsmedicine* 18 (1990): 39–40.

Dalsky, G. P. "Effect of Exercise on Bone: Permissive Influence of Estrogen and Calcium." *Medicine and Science in Sports and Exercise* 22 (1990): 281–285.

DeBenedette, V. "Are Your Patients Exercising Too Much?" *The Physician and Sportsmedicine* 18 (1990): 119–122.

————. "Keeping Pace with the Many Forms of Walking." *The Physician and Sportsmedicine* 16 (1988): 145–150.

Demello, J. J., K. J. Cureton, et al. "Rating of Perceived Exertion at the Lactate Threshold in Trained and Untrained Men and Women." *Medicine and Science in Sports and Exercise* 19 (1987): 354–361.

Dienstbier, R.A. "Behavioral Correlates of Sympathoadrenal Reactivity: the Toughness Model." *Medicine and Science in Sports and Exercise* 23 (1991): 846–851.

Dishman, R. K. "Exercise Compliance: A New View for Public Health." *The Physician and Sportsmedicine* 14 (1986): 127–145.

Dohm, G. L., E. B. Tapscott, and G. J. Kasperek. "Protein Degradation During Endurance, Exercise and Recovery." *Medicine and Science in Sports and Exercise* 19 Suppl. (1987): S166–171.

Drachman, L., and P. Wynne. "Great Grains." New York: Fireside/Simon and Schuster, 1990.

Dressendorfer, R. H., C. E. Wade, and J. H. Scaff. "Increased Morning Heart Rate in Runners: a Valid Sign of Overtraining?" *The Physician and Sportsmedicine* 13 (1985): 77–86.

Duda, M. "The Role of Exercise in Managing Diabetes." *The Physician and Sportsmedicine* 13 (1985): 164–170.

Duncan, J J., J. E. Farr, et al. "The Effects of Aerobic Exercise on Plasma Catecholamines and Blood Pressure in Patients with Mild Essential Hypertension." *Journal of the American Medical Association* 254 (1985): 2609–2613.

Duncan, J. J., N. F. Gordon, and C. B. Scott. "Women Walking for Health and Fitness: How Much Is Enough?" *Journal of the American Medical Association* 266 (1991): 3295–3299.

Dusky, L., and J. J. Leedy. *How to Eat Like a Thin Person.* New York: Simon and Schuster, 1982.

Dustman, R. E., R. O. Ruhling, et al. "Aerobic Exercise Training and Improved Neuropsychological Function of Older Individuals." *Neurobiology of Aging* 5 (1984): 35–42.

Dwyer, J., M. McColgan, et al. "Self-paced Running and the Anaerobic Threshold. (abstr.) *Medicine and Science in Sports and Exercise* 14 (1982): 128.

Ehsani, A. A., T. Ogawa, et al. "Exercise Training Improves Left Ventricular Systolic Function in Older Men." *Circulation* 83 (1991): 96–103.

Elsayed, M., A. H. Ismail, and R. J. Young. "Intellectual Differences of Adult Men Related to Age and Physical Fitness before and after an Exercise Program." *Journal of Gerontology* 35 (1980): 383–387.

Eufemio, M.A. "Calcitonin: Advances in the Therapy of Osteoporosis." *Geriatric Medicine Today* 8 (1989): 106–111.

————. "Vitamin D: Advances in the Therapy of Osteoporosis." *Geriatric Medicine Today* 9 (1990): 37–49.

Evans, W. J., E. C. Fisher, et al. "Protein Metabolism and Endurance Exercise." *The Physician and Sportsmedicine* 11 (1983): 63–72.

Fajans, S. "Maturity-onset Diabetes in Young Black Americans." *New England Journal of Medicine* 317 (1987): 380–381.

Feigley, D. A. "Psychological Burnout in High-level Athletes." *The Physician and Sportsmedicine* 12 (1984): 109–119.

Fellingham, G. W., E. S. Roundy, et al. "Caloric Cost of Walking and Running." *Medicine and Science in Sports and Exercise* 10 (1978): 132–136.

Ferrannini, E., G. Buzzigoli, et al. "Insulin Resistance in Essential Hypertension." *New England Journal of Medicine* 317 (1987): 350–357.

Festinger, L. "Cognitive Dissonance." In *Readings From Scientific American, Contemporary Psychology*, 409–415. San Francisco: W. H. Freeman, 1971.

Fiatarone, M. A., E. C. Marks, et al. "High Intensity Strength Training in Nonagenarians. Effects on Skeletal Muscle." *Journal of the American Medical Association* 263 (1990): 3029–3034.

Finn, J., and R. Morse. "Relationship Between Heart Rate and Perceived Exertion in Multi-mode Exercise for Cardiac Rehabilitation Patients." (abstr.) *Medicine and Science in Sports and Exercise* 22 Suppl. (1990): 56.

Foreyt, J. P. "Diet, Behavior Modification, and Obesity: Nine Questions Most Often Asked by Physicians." *Consultant* 30 (1990): 53–59.

Foreyt, J. P., and G. K. Goodrick. "Factors Common to Successful Therapy for the Obese Patient." *Medicine and Science in Sports and Exercise* 23 (1991): 292–227.

Freundlich, M., G. Zilleruelo, et al. "Infant Formula as a Cause of Aluminum Toxicity in Neonatal Uraemia." *The Lancet* (17 September 1985): 527–529.

Friedman, G. R., M. H. Floch, and M. M. Schuster. "The Dietary Fiber Controversy." *Practical Gastroenterology* 14 (1990): 56–88.

Friedman, R., and R. M. Tappen. "The Effect of Planned Walking on Communication in Alzheimer's Disease." *Journal of the American Geriatric Society* 39 (1991): 650–654.

Frohlich, E. D., ed. "Hypertension 1989: a Symposium." *Practical Cardiology* 15 (1989): 48–96.

Gall, S. L. "Food Groups Pyramid Replaces Pie." *The Physician and Sportsmedicine* 20 (1992): 23.

Goldstein, D. "Clinical Applications for Exercise." *The Physician and Sportsmedicine* 17 (1989): 89.

Gondek, K., P. P. Lamy, and S. M. Speedie. "Medical Expert System: Hypertension in the Elderly." *Geriatric Medicine Today* 9 (1990): 51–54.

Goodwin, G. M., P. J. Cowen, et al. "Plasma Concentrations of Tryptophan and Dieting." *British Medical Journal* 300 (1990): 1499–1500.

Gordon, N. F., J. P. Van Rensburg, et al. "Effect of Dual Beta-blockade and Calcium Antagonism on Endurance Performance." *Medicine and Science in Sports and Exercise* 19 (1987): 1–6.

Gorski, J., L. B. Oscai, and W. Palmer. "Hepatic Lipid Metabolism in Exercise and Training." *Medicine and Science in Sports and Exercise* 22 (1990): 213–219.

Grant, J. C. B. *An Atlas of Anatomy.* Baltimore: Williams and Wilkins, 1947.

Graves, J. E., D. A. Martin, et al. "Physiological Responses to Walking with Hand Weights, Wrist Weights, and Ankle Weights." *Medicine and Science in Sports and Exercise* 20 (1988): 265–271.

Graves, J. E., M. L. Pollack, et al. "The Effect of Hand-held Weights on the Physiological Response to Walking Exercise." *Medicine and Science in Sports and Exercise* 19 (1987): 260–264.

Grundy, S. M. "Comparison of Monounsaturated Fatty Acids and Carbohydrates for Lowering Plasma Cholesterol." *New England Journal of Medicine* 314 (1986): 745–748.

Hage, P. "Behavior Strategies Increase Compliance." *The Physician and Sportsmedicine* 10 (1982): 45.

Hagerman, F. C., R. S. Hikida, et al. "Muscle Damage in Marathon Runners." *The Physician and Sportsmedicine* 12 (1984): 39–48.

Hazzard, W. R. "Why Do Women Live Longer than Men? Biological Differences that Influence Longevity." *Postgraduate Medicine* 85 (1989): 271–283.

Heaney, R. P. "Is Calcium Intake Important for Healthy Bones?" *Osteo News* 1 (1989): 6–7.

Helmrich, S. P., D. R. Ragland, et al. "Physical Activity and Reduced Occurrence of Non insulin Dependent Diabetes Mellitus." *New England Journal of Medicine* 324 (1991): 147–152.

Herbert, W. G., V. F. Froelicher, et al. "Exercise Tests for Coronary and Asymptomatic Patients: Risk Factors and Methods." *The Physician and Sportsmedicine* 19 (1991): 55–62.

Hergenroeder, A. C., M. L. Fiorotto, and W. J. Klish. "Body Composition in Ballet Dancers Measured by Total Body Conductivity." *Medicine and Science in Sports and Exercise* 23 (1991): 528–533.

Herring, J. L., P. A. Mole, et al. "Effect of Suspending Exercise Training on Resting Metabolic Rate in Women." *Medicine and Science in Sports and Exercise* 24 (1992): 59–65.

Hetherington, M., R. Haemel, et al. "Importance of Considering Ventricular Function when Prescribing Exercise after Acute Myocardial Infarction." *American Journal of Cardiology.* 58 (1986): 891–895.

Hetzler, R. K., R. L Seip, et al. "Effect of Exercise Modality on Ratings of Perceived Exertion at Various Lactate Concentrations." *Medicine and Science in Sports and Exercise* 23 (1991): 88–92.

Heywood, J. T., J. Grimm, et al. "Right Ventricular Systolic Function during Exercise Without Significant Coronary Artery Disease." *American Journal of Cardiology* 67 (1991): 681–686.

Hickson, R. C., and S. M. Czerwinski. "Glucocorticoid Antagonism by Exercise and Androgenic-anabolic Steroids." *Medicine and Science in Sports and Exercise* 22 (1990): 331–340.

Hollenbeck, C. B, and A. M. Coulston. "The Role of Dietary Fiber in the Nutritional Management of Diabetes Mellitus." *Practical Cardiology* 13 (1987): 49–58.

Holloszy, J. O. "Exercise, Health and Aging: A Need for More Information." *Medicine and Science in Sports and Exercise* 15 (1983): 1–5.

Hubbard, R. W., and L. E. Armstrong. "Exertional Heatstroke: an International Perspective." *Medicine and Science in Sports and Exercise* 22 (1990): 2–36.

Jackson, A., R. K. Dishman, et al. "The Heart Rate, Perceived Exertion, and Pace of the 1.5 Mile Run." *Medicine and Science in Sports and Exercise* 13 (1981): 224–228.

Jacobs, I. "The Effects of Thermal Dehydration on Performance of the Wingate Anaerobic Test." *International Journal of Sports Medicine* 1 (1980): 21–24.

Jaeger, J. J., E. C. Deal, et al. "Cold Air Inhalation and Esophageal Temperature in Exercising Humans." *Medicine and Science in Sports and Exercise* 12 (1980): 365–369.

Jensen, M. D., and J. M. Miles. "The Roles of Diet and Exercise in the Management of Patients with Insulin-dependent Diabetes Mellitus." *Mayo Clinic Proceedings* 61 (1986): 813–818.

Jesek, J. K., N. B. Martin, et al. "Changes in Plasma Free Fatty Acids and Glycerols during Prolonged Exercise in Trained and Hypertensive Persons Taking Propranolol and Pindolol." *American Journal of Cardiology* 66 (1990): 1336–1340.

Jones, J. G. "Use of Very Low Calorie Diets in Obesity." *American Family Physician* 42 (1990): 1254–1256.

Kappagoda, C. T., and R. Haennel. "Exercise Training of Patients in Cardiac Rehabilitation Programs." *Practical Cardiology* 14 (1988): 69–78.

Kasch, F. W., and J. L. Boyer. "The Effect of Physical Activity and Inactivity on Aerobic Power in Older Men (A Longitudinal Study)." *The Physician and Sportsmedicine* 18 (1990): 73–83.

Kasch, F. W., J. P. Wallace, et al. "A Longitudinal Study of Cardiovascular Stability in Active Men Aged 45 to 65 Years." *The Physician and Sportsmedicine* 16 (1988): 117–26.

Kaufmann, E. "Shoe Biz." *Health* (September 1989): 60–61.

Kern, P. A., J. M. Ong, et al. "The Effects of Weight Loss on the Activity and Expression of Adipose-tissue Lipoprotein Lipase in Very Obese Humans." *New England Journal of Medicine* 32 (1990): 1053–1058.

Ketchum, B. "Why Walking Shoes?" *Walking Magazine* 6 (1991): 4.

Khaw, K. T., and E. Barrett-Connor. "Dietary Potassium and Stroke-associated Mortality: a 12-year Prospective Population Study." *New England Journal of Medicine* 316 (1987): 235–240.

Kleiner, S. M. "Yogurt: a Cultured Cure-all?" *The Physician and Sportsmedicine* 20 (1992): 51–52.

————. "Fiber Facts: How to Fight Disease with a High Fiber Diet." *The Physician and Sportsmedicine* 18 (1990): 19–22.

————. "Seafood and Your Heart." *The Physician and Sportsmedicine* 18 (1990): 19–20.

Koike, A., H. Itoh, M. Doi, et al. "Beat-to-beat Evaluation of Cardiac Function during Recovery from Upright Bicycle Exercise in Patients with Coronary Artery Disease." *American Heart Journal* 120 (1990): 316–323.

Kramsch, D. M., A. J. Aspen, et al. "Reduction of Coronary Atherosclerosis by Moderate Conditioning Exercise in Monkeys on an Atherogenic Diet." *New England Journal of Medicine* 305 (1981): 1483–1488.

Krishna, G. G., and S. C. Kapoor. "Potassium Depletion Exacerbates Essential Hypertension." *Annals of Internal Medicine* 115 (1991): 77–83.

Kriska, A. M., C. Bayles, et al. "A Randomized Exercise Trial in Older Women: Increased Activity over Two Years and the Factors Associated with Compliance." *Medicine and Science in Sports and Exercise* 18 (1986): 557–561.

Kuntzleman, C. T. "Fitness for Life: Exercise Your Way to Better Health." *Blue Cross/Blue Shield Booklet #0451* (1989).

Kupari, M., P. Koskinen, et al. "Left Ventricular Filling Impairment in Asymptomatic Chronic Alcoholics." *American Journal of Cardiology* 66 (1990): 1473–1476.

Kushner, R. F. "Cardiovascular Effects of Extreme Dieting." *Internal Medicine for the Specialist* 11 (1990): 67–77.

La Fontaine, T., B. R. Londeree, et al. "The Effect of Intensity and Quantity of Exercise on the Aerobic and Anaerobic Thresholds" (abstr.). *Medicine and Science in Sports and Exercise* 14 (1982): 127.

Landsberg, L. "Insulin and Hypertension: Lessons from Obesity." *New England Journal of Medicine* 317 (1987): 378–379.

Legwold, G. "Healthy Heart Not Hampered by Aging." *The Physician and Sportsmedicine* 12 (1984): 27.

Levin, S. "Can Older Be Better? The Aging Athlete." *The Physician and Sportsmedicine* 20 (1992): 139–146.

Lindner, P. G., B. R. Bistrian, et al. "The Great Diet Debate (Part I)." *Obesity/Bariatric Medicine* 10 (1981): 36–39.

Lovejoy, C. O. "Evolution of Human Walking." *Scientific American* 264 (1988): 118–125.

Luke, B. *Principles of Nutrition and Diet Therapy.* Boston/Toronto: Little, Brown and Company, 1984.

Macera, C. A., R. R. Pate, et al. "Predicting Lower-extremity Injuries among Habitual Runners." *Archives of Internal Medicine* 149 (1989): 2565–2568.

Mailloux, L. U. "The Necessity for Normalizing Pressure, the Means to Effect It." *Consultant* 32 (1992): 48–54.

Malkin, M. *Walking—The Pleasure Exercise.* Emmaus, PA: Rodale Press, 1986.

Martin, D. W. "Fat Soluble Vitamins," 118–127. In *Harper's Biochemistry, 22/e.* Norwalk/San Mateo: Appleton and Lange, 1990.

———. "Water and Minerals," 649–660. In *Harper's Biochemistry, 22/e.* Norwalk/San Mateo: Appleton and Lange, 1990.

———. "Water Soluble Vitamins," 101–117. In *Harper's Biochemistry, 22/e.* Norwalk/San Mateo: Appleton and Lange, 1990.

Masoro, E. J. "A Physiological Approach to the Study of Aging." *Medical Times* 117 (1989): 63–67.

Massie, B. M. "To Combat Hypertension, Increase Activity." *The Physician and Sportsmedicine* 20 (1992): 89–111.

Mattson, F. H. "A Changing Role for Dietary Monounsaturated Fatty Acids." *Journal of the American Dietetic Association* 89 (1989): 387–391.

Mattson, F. H., and S. M. Grundy. "Comparison of Effects of Dietary Saturated, Monounsaturated, and Polyunsaturated Fatty Acids on Plasma Lipids and Lipoproteins in Man." *Journal of Lipid Research* 26 (1985):194–202.

Mayes, P. A. "Carbohydrates," 147–157. In *Harper's Biochemistry, 22/e.* Norwalk/San Mateo: Appleton and Lange, 1990.

Mayes, P. A. "Lipids," 194–224. In *Harper's Biochemistry, 22/e.* Norwalk/San Mateo: Appleton and Lange, 1990.

McClendon, I. "Honolulu Marathon Clinics Stress Safety, Not Winning." *The Physician and Sportsmedicine* 10 (1982): 153–156.

McDonald, R. B., S. Wickler, et al. "Meal Induced Thermogenesis Following Exercise Training in the Rat." *Medicine and Science in Sports and Exercise* 20 (1988): 44–49.

McFarland, K. F., C. Baker, and S. D. Ferguson. "Demystifying Hypoglycemia: When Is It Real and How Can You Tell?" *Postgraduate Medicine* 82 (1987): 54–68.

Menier, D. R., L. G. C. E. Pugh, "The Relation of Oxygen Intake and Velocity of Walking and Running, in Competition Walkers." *Journal of Physiology* 197 (1968): 717–721.

Miller, M. "Fluid and Electrolyte Balance in the Elderly." *Geriatrics* 42 (1987): 65–76.

Minor, M. A., J. E. Hewett, et al. "Efficacy of Physical Conditioning Exercise in Patients with Rheumatoid Arthritis and Osteoarthritis." *Arthritis and Rheumatism* 32 (1989): 1396–1405.

Mole, P. A., and J. Stern. "Exercise Reverses Depressed Metabolic Rate Produced by Severe Caloric Restriction." *Medicine and Science in Sports and Exercise* 21 (1989): 29–33.

Monahan, T. "Exercise and Depression: Swapping Sweat for Serenity." *The Physician and Sportsmedicine* 14 (1986): 192–197.

———. "From Activity to Eternity." *The Physician and Sportsmedicine* 14 (1986): 156–164.

———. "Perceived Exertion: An Old Exercise Tool Finds New Applications." *The Physician and Sportsmedicine* 16 (1988): 174–179.

Moore-Ede, M. C., C. A. Czeisler, and G. S. Richardson. "Circadian Timekeeping in Health and Disease." *New England Journal of Medicine* 309 (1983): 469–475.

Morgan, W. P. "Affective Beneficence of Vigorous Physical Activity." *Medicine and Science in Sports and Exercise* 17 (1985): 94-100.

Munnings, F. "Exercise: Is Any Time the Prime Time?" *The Physician and Sportsmedicine* 19 (1991): 101–104.

Murray, M. P., G. N. Guten, et al. "Kinematic and Electromyographic Patterns of Olympic Racewalkers." *American Journal of Sports Medicine* 11 (1983): 68–74.

Nash, H. L. "Exercising the Body to Sharpen the Mind." *The Physician and Sportsmedicine* 14 (1986): 34.

National Asthma Education Program: Expert Panel Report. "Executive Summary: Guidelines for the Diagnosis and Management of Asthma." U.S. Department of Health and Human Services, PHS, NIH (1991).

Nelson, L., M. D. Esler, et al. "Effect of Changing Levels of Physical Activity on Blood Pressure and Haemodynamics in Essential Hypertension." *The Lancet* (30 August 1986): 473–476.

Nelson, R. A. "Nutrition and Physical Performance." *The Physician and Sportsmedicine* 10 (1982): 55–63.

Nicholson, J. P., and D. B. Case. "Carboxyhemoglobin Levels in New York City Runners." *The Physician and Sportsmedicine* 11 (1983): 135-138.

Noble, B. J., G. A. Borg, et al. "A Category-ratio Perceived Exertion Scale: Relationship to Blood and Muscle Lactates and Heart Rate." *Medicine and Science in Sports and Exercise* 15 (1983): 523–528.

O'Toole, M. L., W. B. D. Hiler, et al. "Hemolysis during Triathlon Races: Its Relation to Race Distance." *Medicine and Science in Sports and Exercise* 20 (1988): 272–275.

Oldridge, N. B., and D. L. Streiner. "The Health Belief Model: Predicting Compliance and Dropout in Cardiac Rehabilitation." *Medicine and Science in Sports and Exercise* 22 (1990): 678–683.

Ornish, D. "Lessons from the Lifestyle Heart Trial." *Choices in Cardiology* 5 (1991): 24–27.

Ornish, D., S. E. Brown, et al. "Can Lifestyle Changes Reverse Coronary Heart Disease?" *The Lancet* 336 (1990): 129–133.

Oscai, L. B. "Preface to Exercise and Triacylglycerol Metabolism." *Medicine and Science in Sports and Exercise* 15 (1983): 330.

Othersen, M. "Health Watch: Heart Rate, New Math." *Runners World* (August 1991): 18.

Pacelli, L. C. "Straight Talk on Posture." *The Physician and Sportsmedicine* 19 (1991): 124–127.

Pacini, G., and F. Beccaro. "Reduced Beta-cell Secretion and Insulin Hepatic Extraction in Healthy Elderly Subjects." *Journal of the American Geriatric Society* 38 (1991): 1283–1289.

Pak, C. Y. C. "Calcium Metabolism." *Journal of the American College of Nutrition* 8 (1985): 465–535.

Palank, E. A., and E. H. Hargreaves. "The Benefits of Walking the Golf Course." *The Physician and Sportsmedicine* 18 (1990): 77–80.

Palmer, W. K. "Hormonal Regulation of Myocardial Lipolysis." *Medicine and Science in Sports and Exercise* 15 (1983): 331–335.

Pedersen, O., H. Beck-Nielsen, and L. Heding. "Increased Insulin Receptors after Exercise in Patients with Insulin-dependent Diabetes Mellitus." *New England Journal of Medicine* 302 (1980): 886–891.

Peronnet, F., G. Thibault, et al. "Correlation Between Ventilatory Threshold and Endurance Capability in Marathon Runners." *Medicine and Science in Sports and Exercise* 19 (1987): 610–615.

Perruse, L., A. Tremblay, et al. "Genetic and Environmental Influences on Level of Habitual Physical Activity and Exercise Participation." *American Journal of Epidemiology* 129 (1989): 1012–1022.

Peterson, S. E., and M. D. Peterson. "Muscle Strength and Bone Density with Weight Training in Middle-aged Women." *Medicine and Science in Sports and Exercise* 23 (1991): 499–504.

Pierron, R. L., H. M. Perry, et al. "The Aging Hip." *Journal of the American Geriatric Society* 38 (1990): 1339–1352.

Podsiadlo, D., and S. Richardson. "The timed 'up and go': A Test of Basic Functional Mobility for Frail Elderly Persons." *Journal of the American Geriatric Society* 39 (1991): 142–148.

Pollack, M.L., J. F. Carroll, et al. "Injuries and Adherence to Walk/jog and Resistance Training Programs in the Elderly." *Medicine and Science in Sports and Exercise* 22 (1991): 1194–1200.

Pollock, M. L., H. S. Miller, Jr., et al. "Effects of Walking on Body Composition and Cardiovascular Function of Middle Aged Men. *Journal of Applied Physiology* 30 (1971):126–130.

Porcari, J., R. McCarron, et al. "Is Fast Walking an Adequate Aerobic Training Stimulus?" *The Physician and Sportsmedicine* 15 (1987): 119–129.

Porter, K. "Psychologic Characteristics of the Average Female Runner." *The Physician and Sportsmedicine* 13 (1985): 171–175.

Powell, K. E., H. W. Kohl, et al. "An Epidemiological Perspective on the Causes of Running Injuries." *The Physician and Sportsmedicine* 14 (1986): 100–114.

Practical Pointers. "Ski Pole Support." *Consultant* 29 (1989): 35.

Preston, J. A., and S. M. Retchin. "The Management of Geriatric Hypertension in Health Maintenance Organizations." *Journal of the American Geriatric Society* 39 (1991): 683–690.

Prince, R. L., M. Smith, et al. "Prevention of Postmenopausal Osteoporosis: A Comparative Study of Exercise, Calcium Supplementation, and Hormone-replacement Therapy." *New England Journal of Medicine* 325 (1991): 1189–1195.

Raglin, J. S., W. P. Morgan, et al. "Mood and Self-motivation in Successful and Unsuccessful Female Rowers." *Medicine and Science in Sports and Exercise* 22 (1990): 849–853.

Raisz, L. G. "Local and Systemic Factors in the Pathogenesis of Osteoporosis." *New England Journal of Medicine* 318 (1988): 818–825.

Ramsey, M. L. "Managing Friction Blisters of the Feet." *The Physician and Sportsmedicine* 20 (1992):117–124.

Ready, A. E., and H. A. Quinney. "Alterations in Anaerobic Threshold as the Result of Endurance Training and Detraining." *Medicine and Science in Sports and Exercise* 14 (1982): 292–296.

Reed, R. L., K. Yochum, et al. "The Interrelationship between Physical Exercise, Muscle Strength and Body Adiposity in a Healthy, Elderly Population." *Journal of the American Geriatric Society* 39 (1991): 1189–1193.

Reginster, J. Y., and A. Albert. "1-year Controlled Randomized Trial of Prevention of Early Postmenopausal Bone Loss with Intranasal Calcitonin." *The Lancet* (26 December 1987): 1481–1483.

Rhymes, J. A. "Can You Correct Your Patient's Gait Disorder?" *Senior Patient* (December 1990): 36–40.

Riggs, B. L. "A New Option for Treating Osteoporosis." *New England Journal of Medicine* 323 (1990): 124–125.

Rives, David A. *Walk Yourself Thin.* Ventura, CA: Moon River, 1990.

Robbins, D. C., and S. Carleton. "Managing the Diabetic Athlete." *The Physician and Sportsmedicine* 17 (1989): 45–54.

Robbins, S. E., and G. J. Gouw. "Athletic Footwear: Unsafe Due to Percep-tual Illusions." *Medicine and Science in Sports and Exercise* 23 (1991): 217–224.

Robertson, L., C. Flinders, and B. Ruppenthal. "The New Laurel's Kitchen." Berkeley, CA: Ten Speed Press, 1986.

Robertson, R. J., J. E. Falkel, et al. "Effect of Blood pH on Peripheral and Central Signals of Perceived Exertion." *Medicine and Science in Sports and Exercise* 18 (1986): 114–122.

Robinson, G. "Where's the Beef?" *Main Event* 5 (1990): 41–43.

Rodwell, V. "Biosynthesis of Amino Acids," 275–276. In *Harper's Biochem-istry, 22/e*. Norwalk/San Mateo: Appleton and Lange, 1990.

———. "Catabolism of Amino Acid Nitrogen," 273–279. In *Harper's Bio-chemistry, 22/e*. Norwalk/San Mateo: Appleton and Lange, 1990.

Rogers, C. C. "Fitness May be a Woman's Best Friend." *The Physician and Sportsmedicine* 12 (1984): 146–156.

Rogers, M. A., G. A. Stull, and F. S. Apple. "Creatine Kinase Isoenzyme Activities in Men and Women following a Marathon Race." *Medicine and Sci-ence in Sports and Exercise* 17 (1985): 679–682.

Rogers, R. L., J. S. Meyer, and K. F. Mortel. "After Reaching Retirement Age, Physical Activity Sustains Cerebral Perfusion and Cognition." *Journal of the American Geriatric Society* 38 (1990): 123–128.

Roos, R. "Warm Muscles Are Less Likely to Tear." *The Physician and Sportsmedicine* 17 (1989): 24.

Rose, C. P., and D. Bailey. "Injuries in Athletes Outside Their NCAA Sports." *The Physician and Sportsmedicine* 11 (1983): 103–105.

Roubenoff, R. A. "Calorie Requirements for Weight Loss." *Choices in Cardiol-ogy* 3 (1989): 169–172.

———. "Hypocholesterolemic Effects of Oat Bran and Legumes." *Choices In Cardiology* 4 (1990): 54–58.

———. "Obesity and Coronary Heart Disease: Clinical Evaluation." *Choices in Cardiology* 5 (1991): 37–40.

———. "Omega-3 Fatty Acids and Coronary Heart Disease." *Choices in Car-diology* 4 (1990): 297–298.

Sager, K. "Senior Fitness—For the Health of It." *The Physician and Sports-medicine* 11 (1983): 31–36.

Scanning Sports. *The Physician and Sportsmedicine* 20 (1992): 2.

Schmid, J. "Fit Feet." *Vogue* (June 1987): 246, 268.

Schocken, D. D., and J. A. Blumenthal. "Left Ventricular and Psychological Response to Exercise Training in Older Patients." *Primary Cardiology* 11 (1985): 64–74.

Scholfield, D. J., S. Reiser, et al. "Dietary Copper, Simple Sugars, and Metabolic Changes in Pigs." *Journal of Nutritional Biochemistry* 1 (1990): 362–370.

Schorr, I. "Slip Sliding Away: Getting Smart about Fats and Oils." *Walking Magazine* 6 (1991): 28–33.

Scrimgeour, A. G., and J. T. Devlin. "Prescribing Exercise for Patients with IDDM." *Internal Medicine for the Specialist* 12 (1991): 56–70.

Sedlock, D. A., J. A. Fissinger, et al. "Effect of Exercise Intensity and Duration on Postexercise Energy Expenditure." *Medicine and Science in Sports and Exercise* 21 (1989): 662–666.

Sheehan, G. A. "Case of Mumpsimus." *The Physician and Sportsmedicine* 14 (1990): 69.

———. "Fulfilling Our Destiny." *The Physician and Sportsmedicine* 12 (1984): 39.

———. "How Important Is the Clock?" *The Physician and Sportsmedicine,* 12 (1984): 47.

———. "Less Is More." *The Physician and Sportsmedicine* 19 (1991): 21.

———. "Peaking for Life." *The Physician and Sportsmedicine* 10 (1982): 32.

———. "Running Is Not Enough." *The Physician and Sportsmedicine* 13 (1985): 41.

———. "Sports Medicine Renaissance." *The Physician and Sportsmedicine* 18 (1990): 26.

———. "The Best Therapy." *The Physician and Sportsmedicine* 11 (1983): 43.

———. "The Unapproved Drug." *The Physician and Sportsmedicine* 11 (1983): 37.

———. "Think New Thoughts." *The Physician and Sportsmedicine* 16 (1988): 28.

Sheetty, T. W. "Zinc Deficiency and Toxicity." *Internal Medicine for the Specialist* 11 (1990): 132–145.

Shellock, F. G. "Physiological Benefits of Warm-up." *The Physician and Sportsmedicine* 11 (1983): 134–139.

Shephard, R. J. *Ischaemic Heart Disease and Exercise.* Chicago: Yearbook Medical Publishers, 1981.

Shephard, R. J. "Motivation: the Key to Fitness Compliance." *The Physician and Sportsmedicine* 13 (1985): 88–101.

Sherwood, D. E., and D. J. Selder. "Cardiorespiratory Health Reaction Time and Aging." *Medicine and Science in Sports and Exercise* 11 (1979): 186–189.

Sidney, K. H., and R. J. Shephard. "Frequency and Intensity of Exercise Training for Elderly Subjects." *Medicine and Science in Sports and Exercise* 10 (1978): 125–131.

Siegel, A. J. "Exercise and Diabetes Mellitus: Benefits and Risks." *Your Patient and Fitness* 2 (1988): 6–11.

———. "Postexercise Muscle Cramps and Soreness." *Your Patient and Fitness* 3 (1989): 6–11.

Siep, R. L., D. Snead, et al. "Perceptual Responses and Blood Lactate Concentration: Effect of Training State." *Medicine and Science in Sports and Exercise* 23 (1991): 80–87.

Singer, R. N. "Thought Processes and Emotions in Sport." *The Physician and Sportsmedicine* 10 (1982): 75–88.

Slavin, J. L. "Calcium and Healthy Bones." *The Physician and Sportsmedicine* 13 (1985): 179–181.

Slavin, J. L., G. Lanners, and M. A. Engstrom. "Amino Acid Supplements: Beneficial or Risky?" *The Physician and Sportsmedicine* 16 (1988): 221–224.

Sly, R. M. "History of Exercise Induced Asthma." *Medicine and Science in Sports and Exercise* 18 (1986): 314–317.

Smiley, K. *The Importance of Walking.* New Paltz, NY: Mohonk Lake,1986.

Smith, E. L., and C. Gilligan. "Physical Activity Prescription for the Older Adult." *The Physician and Sportsmedicine* 11 (1983): 91–101.

Smith, E., W. Reddan, and P. E. Smith. "Physical Activity and Calcium Modalities for Bone Mineral Increase in Aged Women." *Medicine and Science in Sports and Exercise* 13 (1981): 60–64.

Smith, M. L., D. L. Hudson, et al. "Exercise Training Bradycardia: The Role of Autonomic Balance." *Medicine and Science in Sports and Exercise* 21 (1989): 40–44.

Somers, V. K., and J. Conway. "Effects of Endurance Training on Baroreflex Sensitivity and Blood Pressure in Borderline Hypertension." *The Lancet* 337 (1991): 1363–1367.

Souominen, H., E. Heikkinen, and T. Parkatti. "Effect of Eight Weeks' Physical Training on Muscle and Connective Tissue of the M. Vastus Lateralis in 69-year-old Men and Women." *Journal of Gerontology* 32 (1977): 33–37.

Stamford, B. "Exercise and Longevity." *The Physician and Sportsmedicine* 12 (1984): 209.

———. "Exercise, Appetite, and Holiday Temptation." *The Physician and Sportsmedicine* 13 (1985): 115.

———. "How Exercise Effects Your Blood Sugar." *The Physician and Sportsmedicine* 19 (1991): 139–140.

———. "Meals and the Timing of Exercise." *The Physician and Sportsmedicine* 17 (1989): 151.

———. "So You Hate to Run." *The Physician and Sportsmedicine* 18 (1990): 175.

———. "What Happened to Old Fashioned Calisthenics?" *The Physician and Sportsmedicine* 13 (1985): 149.

————. "What Is Interval Training?" *The Physician and Sportsmedicine* 17 (1989): 193.

————. "What Is Target Heart Rate?" *The Physician and Sportsmedicine* 15 (1987): 214.

————. "When to Eat and Exercise." *The Physician and Sportsmedicine* 16 (1988): 184.

Stein, J. "Highlights of the Third International Symposium on Osteoporosis. Copenhagen, Denmark. October 14–18, 1990." *Geriatric Medicine Today* 10 (1991): 70–71.

Stewert, E. "Nutrition Management for Exercising Diabetics." *Your Patient and Fitness* 2 (1988): 15–17.

Stillman, R. J., and T. G. Lohman. "Physical Activity and Bone Mineral Content in Women Aged 30–85 Years." *Medicine and Science in Sports and Exercise* 18 (1986): 576–580.

Stone, M. H. "Muscle Conditioning and Muscle Injuries." *Medicine and Science in Sports and Exercise* 22 (1990): 457–462.

Stratton, R., D. P. Wilson, and R. K. Endres. "Acute Glycemic Effects of Exercise in Adolescents with Insulin Dependent Diabetes Mellitus." *The Physician and Sportsmedicine* 16 (1988): 150–157.

Strauss, R. H. "Take a Walk." *The Physician and Sportsmedicine* 14 (1986): 23.

Stromberg, B. V. "Wound Healing in the Elderly." *Geriatric Medicine Today* 8 (1989): 93–97.

Strovas, J. "90-year-olds Increase Strength Dramatically." *The Physician and Sportsmedicine* 18 (1990): 26.

Stunkard, A. J., J. R. Harris, et al. "The Body Mass Index of Twins Who Have Been Reared Apart." *New England Journal of Medicine* 322 (1990): 1483–1487.

Sullivan, J. L. "Stored Iron and Ischemic Heart Disease: Empirical Support for a New Paradigm." *Circulation* 86 (1992): 1036–1037.

Superko, H. R. "Exercise Training, Serum Lipids, and Lipoprotein Particles: Is There a Change Threshold?" *Medicine and Science in Sports and Exercise* 23 (1991): 667–685.

Sussman, A., and R. Goode. *The Magic of Walking.* New York: Simon and Schuster, 1987.

Svensson, B. G, A. Nilsson, et al. "Exposure to Dioxins and Dibenzofurans through the Consumption of Fish." *New England Journal of Medicine* 324 (1991): 8–12.

Tajfel, H. "Experiments in Intergroup Discrimination," 416–422. In *Readings From Scientific American: Contemporary Psychology.* San Francisco: W. H. Freeman and Co., 1971.

Tanji, J. L. "Hypertension, Part I: How Exercise Helps." *The Physician and Sportsmedicine* 18 (1990): 77–82.

Taylor, P., A. Ward, and J. M. Rippe. "Exercising to Health, How Much? How Soon? *The Physician and Sportsmedicine* 19 (1991): 95–104.

Terjung, R. L., B. G. Mackie, et al. "Influence of Exercise on Chylomicron Triacylglycerol Metabolism: Plasma Turnover and Muscle Intake." *Medicine and Science in Sports and Exercise* 15 (1983): 340–347.

Thomas, D. P. "Effects of Acute and Chronic Exercise on Myocardial Ultrastructure." *Medicine and Science in Sports and Exercise* 17 (1985): 546–553.

Thomas, P. "More Studies Back Potassium Use." *Medical World News* (12 June 1989): 30.

Thompson, D. A., L. A. Wolfe, et al. "Acute Effects of Exercise Intensity on Appetite in Young Men." *Medicine and Science in Sports and Exercise* 20 (1988): 222–227.

Thompson, N. N., and C. Foster. "Prediction of Exercise Training Intensity Using Rating of Perceived Exertion" (abstr.). *Medicine and Science in Sports and Exercise* 22 suppl. (1990): S2 (10).

Trials of Hypertension Presentation Collaborative Research Group. "The Effects of Non-pharmacologic Interventions on Blood Pressure of Persons with High Normal Levels: Result of the Trials of Hypertension Prevention, Phase I." *Journal of the American Medical Association* 267 (1992): 1213–1220.

Tutko, T. A., and J. W. Richards. *Motivation. in Psychology of Coaching*. Boston: Allyn and Bacon, 1971.

Van Camp, S. P., and J. L. Boyer. "Cardiovascular Aspects of Aging (part 1)." *The Physician and Sportsmedicine* 17 (1989): 121–130.

Van Camp, S. P. "Prevention of Cardiovascular Complications of Exercise Training." *Practical Cardiology* 14 (1988): 31–46.

Van Gaal, L. F., and M. F. Vandewoude. "Abdominal Fat: Risk Factor for Cardiovascular Disease in the Elderly Diabetic Patient." *Geriatric Medicine Today* 9 (1990): 63–.

Van Vlaanderen, E. "How Low Should Blood Pressure Go?" *Cortlandt Forum* (April 1992): 226–236.

———. "Insulin Resistence: a New Factor in Hypertension?" *Cortlandt Forum* 5 (1992): 178–195.

Walk USA Catalogue. (Spring 1993).

Walking Magazine editors. "Politics of Walking." *Walking Magazine* 2 (1987): 14.

Warner, J. G., I. H. Ullrich, et al. "Combined Effects of Aerobic Exercise and Omega-3 Fatty Acids in Hyperlipedemic Persons." *Medicine and Science in Sports and Exercise* 21 (1989): 498–505.

Watts, N. B., S. T. Harris, et al. "Intermittent Cyclical Etidronate Treatment of Postmenopausal Osteoporosis." *New England Journal of Medicine* 323 (1990): 73–79.

Weltman, A., and B. Stamford. "Psychological Effects of Exercise." *The Physician and Sportsmedicine* 11 (1983): 175.

Wenger, N. K. "Home vs. Supervised Exercise Training after M.I." *Practical Cardiology* 15 (1989): 47–53.

Whalen, R. T., D. R. Carter, and C. R. Steele. "Influence of Physical Activity on the Regulation of Bone Density." *Journal of Biomechanics* 21 (1988): 825–837.

White, S. C., and D. Winter. "Mechanical Power Analysis of Lower Limb Musculature in Racewalking." *International Journal of Sport Biomechanics* 1 (1985): 15–24.

Wilmore, J. H. "Thunder Thighs and Love Handles." *Sports Medicine Digest* 12 (1990): 1–2.

Zeppilli, P. "The Athlete's Heart: a Differentiation of Training Effects from Organic Heart Disease." *Practical Cardiology* 14 (1988): 61–84.

Zevin, D. "Brother Isadore: Footloose Friar." *Walking Magazine* 4 (1989): 9.

———. "Indiana Freys: It's All in the Family." *Walking Magazine* 5 (1990): 8.

———. "Walk on the Wild Side." *Walking Magazine* 2 (1987): 18–19.

———. "Walking Away from Arthritis." *Walking Magazine* 5 (1990): 15.

———. "Warming Up to Exercise." *Walking Magazine* 6 (1991): 23.

Index